Special Techniques and Technical Advances in PET/CT Imaging

Editor

RAKESH KUMAR

PET CLINICS

www.pet.theclinics.com

Consulting Editor
ABASS ALAVI

January 2016 • Volume 11 • Number 1

ELSEVIER

1600 John F. Kennedy Boulevard • Suite 1800 • Philadelphia, Pennsylvania, 19103-2899

http://www.pet.theclinics.com

PET CLINICS Volume 11, Number 1
January 2016 ISSN 1556-8598, ISBN-13: 978-0-323-41462-3

Editor: John Vassallo (j.vassallo@elsevier.com)
Developmental Editor: Meredith Clinton

PET Clinics (ISSN 1556-8598) is published quarterly by Elsevier Inc., 360 Park Avenue South, New York, NY 10010-1710. Months of issue are January, April, July, and October. Periodicals postage paid at New York, NY, and additional mailing offices. Subscription prices per year are $225.00 (US individuals), $366.00 (US institutions), $100.00 (US students), $255.00 (Canadian individuals), $412.00 (Canadian institutions), $140.00 (Canadian students), $260.00 (foreign individuals), $412.00 (foreign institutions), and $140.00 (foreign students). To receive student and resident rate, orders must be accompanied by name of affiliated institution, date of term, and the signature of program/residency coordinator on institution letterhead. Orders will be billed at individual rate until proof of status is received. Foreign air speed delivery is included in all Clinics subscription prices. All prices are subject to change without notice. POSTMASTER: Send address changes to PET Clinics, Elsevier Health Sciences Division, Subscription Customer Service, 3251 Riverport Lane, Maryland Heights, MO 63043. **Customer Service: 1-800-654-2452 (U.S. and Canada); 314-447-8871 (outside U.S. and Canada). Fax: 314-447-8029. E-mail: journalscustomerservice-usa@elsevier.com (for print support);** journalsonlinesupport-usa@elsevier.com **(for online support).**

Reprints. For copies of 100 or more of articles in this publication, please contact the Commercial Reprints Department, Elsevier Inc., 360 Park Avenue South, New York, NY 10010-1710. Tel.: 212-633-3874; Fax: 212-633-3820; E-mail: reprints@elsevier.com.

PET Clinics is covered in MEDLINE/PubMed (Index Medicus).

Contributors

CONSULTING EDITOR

ABASS ALAVI, MD, PhD (Hon), Dsc (Hon)
Professor of Radiology, Division of Nuclear
Medicine, Department of Radiology, University
of Pennsylvania School of Medicine, Hospital
of the University of Pennsylvania, Philadelphia,
Pennsylvania

EDITOR

RAKESH KUMAR, MD, PhD
Professor and Head, Diagnostic Nuclear
Medicine Division, Department of Nuclear
Medicine, All India Institute of Medical
Sciences, New Delhi, India

AUTHORS

KRISHAN KANT AGARWAL, MD
Diagnostic Nuclear Medicine Division,
Department of Nuclear Medicine, All India
Institute of Medical Sciences, New Delhi,
India

ABASS ALAVI, MD, PhD (Hon), Dsc (Hon)
Professor of Radiology, Division of Nuclear
Medicine, Department of Radiology, University
of Pennsylvania School of Medicine, Hospital
of the University of Pennsylvania, Philadelphia,
Pennsylvania

MATEOS BOGONI, MD
Quanta Diagnóstico e Terapia, Diagnostic and
Therapy Clinic, Curitiba, Paraná, Brazil

JULIANO J. CERCI, PhD
Quanta Diagnóstico e Terapia, Diagnostic and
Therapy Clinic, Curitiba, Paraná, Brazil

ANIL CHAUHAN, MD
Assistant Professor, Division of Abdominal
Imaging, Department of Radiology,
University of Pennsylvania, Philadelphia,
Pennsylvania

CHANDAN J. DAS, MD
Assistant Professor, Department of Radiology,
All India Institute of Medical Sciences, New
Delhi, India

VARUN SINGH DHULL, MBBS, MD
Department of Nuclear Medicine, All India
Institute of Medical Sciences, New Delhi,
India

MITSUKAZU GOTOH, MD, PhD
Chairman of Surgery, Chest Surgery, School
of Medicine, Fukushima Medical University,
Fukushima, Japan

PETER GRUPE, MD
Department of Nuclear Medicine, Odense
University Hospital, Odense, Denmark

ARUN K. GUPTA, MD
Department of Radiology, All India Institute of
Medical Sciences, New Delhi, India

RAMEZ HANNA, MD
Division of Abdominal Imaging, Department of
Radiology, University of Pennsylvania,
Philadelphia, Pennsylvania

MITSUNORI HIGUCHI, MD, PhD
Chest Surgery, School of Medicine, Fukushima
Medical University, Fukushima, Japan

POUL FLEMMING HØILUND-CARLSEN, MD, DMSc
Department of Nuclear Medicine, Odense
University Hospital, Odense, Denmark

SINA HOUSHMAND, MD
Department of Radiology, University of
Pennsylvania, Philadelphia, Pennsylvania

LISA P. JONES, MD, PhD
Division of Abdominal Imaging, Department of
Radiology, University of Pennsylvania,
Philadelphia, Pennsylvania

RAKESH KUMAR, MD, PhD
Professor and Head, Diagnostic Nuclear
Medicine Division, Department of Nuclear
Medicine, All India Institute of Medical
Sciences, New Delhi, India

SMITA MANCHANDA, MD
Department of Radiology, All India Institute of
Medical Sciences, New Delhi, India

BHAGWANT RAI MITTAL, MD
Department of Nuclear Medicine, Post
Graduate Institute of Medical Education and
Research, Chandigarh, India

ANIRBAN MUKHERJEE, MD
Diagnostic Nuclear Medicine Division,
Department of Nuclear Medicine, All India
Institute of Medical Sciences, New Delhi,
India

AFTAB HASAN NAZAR, MBBS, MD
Department of Nuclear Medicine, All India
Institute of Medical Sciences, New Delhi, India

ANANYA PANDA, MD
Department of Radiology, All India Institute of
Medical Sciences, New Delhi, India

NEELIMA RANA, MBBS, MD
Department of Radiodiagnosis, MS Ramaiah
Medical College, Bengaluru, India

SHAMBO GUHA ROY, MD
Diagnostic Nuclear Medicine Division,
Department of Nuclear Medicine, All India
Institute of Medical Sciences, New Delhi, India

ALI SALAVATI, MD, MPH
Department of Radiology, University of
Pennsylvania, Philadelphia, Pennsylvania;
Department of Radiology, University of
Minnesota, Minneapolis, Minnesota

EIVIND ANTONSEN SEGTNAN, BSc
Department of Nuclear Medicine, Odense
University Hospital, Odense, Denmark

ANSHUL SHARMA, MD
Department of Nuclear Medicine, All India
Institute of Medical Sciences, New Delhi, India

HIROYUKI SUZUKI, MD, PhD
Chest Surgery, School of Medicine, Fukushima
Medical University, Fukushima, Japan

ELENA TABACCHI, MD
Nuclear Medicine Unit, S. Orsola-Malpighi
Hospital, Bologna, Italy

Contents

urinary tract activity. Intense radiotracer activity in urinary tract interferes in image interpretation and leads to false-negative results in diagnosis and detection of local recurrence and regional lymph node metastases. It is imperative to minimize unnecessary urinary bladder activity to improve the diagnostic yield of PET/CT. All the techniques described in the literature have their pros and cons. This article discusses FDG PET/CT in evaluation of urinary bladder cancer, cervical cancer, and ovarian cancer.

Radiofrequency ablation (RFA) is a useful tool for local control of unresectable pulmonary neoplastic lesions; however, RFA is limited to tumors smaller than 4 cm and peripheral lesions. The sensitivity and specificity of FDG-PET are higher than those of computed tomography. FDG-PET at 3 to 6 months after RFA is important for predicting recurrence. Complications associated with RFA, such as infection and abscess formation, which concentrate glucose in the ablation area, can cause false-positive findings in PET examination. Knowledge of the morphologic imaging features of these complications is important in avoiding these potential pitfalls.

PET/computed tomography (CT) combines the anatomic information from CT with PET metabolic characterization. 18F-fluorodeoxyglucose (FDG) PET is helpful to differentiate malignant lesions from benign ones, that usually show lower or no uptake. However, active inflammation or infectious disease might also present FDG uptake. Studies confirm the great value of PET/CT as the imaging method of choice for guiding biopsy procedures. Novel PET radiopharmaceuticals are also being investigated for guiding biopsies.

The techniques of dual-time-point imaging (DTPI) and delayed-time-point imaging, which are mostly being used for distinction between inflammatory and malignant diseases, has increased the specificity of fluorodeoxyglucose (FDG)-PET for diagnosis and prognosis of certain diseases. A gradually increasing trend of FDG uptake over time has been shown in malignant cells, and a decreasing or constant trend has been shown in inflammatory/infectious processes. Tumor heterogeneity can be assessed by using early and delayed imaging because differences between primary versus metastatic sites become more detectable compared with single time points. This article discusses the applications of DTPI and delayed-time-point imaging.

Is there a need for the contrast-enhanced PET/computed tomography (CT) scan or is the low-dose, non-contrast-enhanced PET/CT scan sufficient? The topic has been debated time and again. Although low-dose noncontrast CT serves the purpose of simple anatomic correlation and attenuation correction of PET images, many times patients have to undergo additional contrast-enhanced diagnostic imaging modalities, which may lead to a delay in decision-making. In this review, the authors have addressed various such issues related to the use of contrast agents and special techniques of clinical interest based on their utility in dual-modality PET/CT.

PET CLINICS

THE CLINICS ARE AVAILABLE ONLINE!
Access your subscription at:
www.theclinics.com

PROGRAM OBJECTIVE

The goal of the *PET Clinics* is to keep practicing radiologists and radiology residents up to date with current clinical practice in positron emission tomography by providing timely articles reviewing the state of the art in patient care.

TARGET AUDIENCE

Practicing radiologists, radiology residents, and other health care professionals who provide patient care utilizing radiologic findings.

LEARNING OBJECTIVES

Upon completion of this activity, participants will be able to:
1. Review special techniques in imaging for cancers, such as those of head and neck, and malignant tumors.
2. Discuss the uses of contrast media and imaging-based intervention in clinical practice.
3. Recognize recent advances in imaging for illnesses other than cancers.

ACCREDITATION

The Elsevier Office of Continuing Medical Education (EOCME) is accredited by the Accreditation Council for Continuing Medical Education (ACCME) to provide continuing medical education for physicians.

The EOCME designates this enduring material for a maximum of 15 *AMA PRA Category 1 Credit*(s)™. Physicians should claim only the credit commensurate with the extent of their participation in the activity.

All other health care professionals requesting continuing education credit for this enduring material will be issued a certificate of participation.

DISCLOSURE OF CONFLICTS OF INTEREST

The EOCME assesses conflict of interest with its instructors, faculty, planners, and other individuals who are in a position to control the content of CME activities. All relevant conflicts of interest that are identified are thoroughly vetted by EOCME for fair balance, scientific objectivity, and patient care recommendations. EOCME is committed to providing its learners with CME activities that promote improvements or quality in healthcare and not a specific proprietary business or a commercial interest.

The planning committee, staff, authors and editors listed below have identified no financial relationships or relationships to products or devices they or their spouse/life partner have with commercial interest related to the content of this CME activity:
Krishan Kant Agarwal, MD; Abass Alavi, MD, PhD (Hon), Dsc (Hon); Mateos Bogoni, MD; Juliano J. Cerci, PhD; Anil Chauhan, MD; Chandan J. Das, MD; Varun Singh Dhull, MBBS, MD; Anjali Fortna; Mitsukazu Gotoh, MD, PhD; Peter Grupe, MD; Arun K. Gupta, MD; Ramez Hanna, MD; Mitsunori Higuchi, MD, PhD; Poul Flemming Høilund-Carlsen, MD, DMSc; Sina Houshmand, MD; Lisa P. Jones, MD, PhD; Rakesh Kumar, MD, PhD; Smita Manchanda, MD; Bhagwant Rai Mittal, MD; Anirban Mukherjee, MD; Aftab Hasan Nazar, MBBS, MD; Mahalakshmi Narayanan; Ananya Panda, MD; Neelima Rana, MBBS, MD; Erin Scheckenbach; Shambo Guha Roy, MD; Ali Salavati, MD, MPH; Eivind Antonsen Segtnan, BSc; Anshul Sharma, MD; Hiroyuki Suzuki, MD, PhD; Elena Tabacchi, MD; John Vassallo.

UNAPPROVED/OFF-LABEL USE DISCLOSURE

The EOCME requires CME faculty to disclose to the participants:
1. When products or procedures being discussed are off-label, unlabelled, experimental, and/or investigational (not US Food and Drug Administration [FDA] approved); and
2. Any limitations on the information presented, such as data that are preliminary or that represent ongoing research, interim analyses, and/or unsupported opinions. Faculty may discuss information about pharmaceutical agents that is outside of FDA-approved labelling. This information is intended solely for CME and is not intended to promote off-label use of these medications. If you have any questions, contact the medical affairs department of the manufacturer for the most recent prescribing information.

TO ENROLL

To enroll in the PET Clinics Continuing Medical Education program, call customer service at 1-800-654-2452 or sign up online at http://www.theclinics.com/home/cme. The CME program is available to subscribers for an additional annual fee of USD $235.

METHOD OF PARTICIPATION

In order to claim credit, participants must complete the following:
1. Complete enrolment as indicated above.
2. Read the activity.
3. Complete the CME Test and Evaluation. Participants must achieve a score of 70% on the test. All CME Tests and Evaluations must be completed online.

CME INQUIRIES/SPECIAL NEEDS

For all CME inquiries or special needs, please contact elsevierCME@elsevier.com.

Preface

Special Techniques and Technical Advances in PET/ Computed Tomographic Imaging

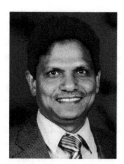

Rakesh Kumar, MD, PhD
Editor

Functional imaging, in particular, PET, is a unique imaging tool showing both molecular function and metabolic activity information that are not available with other modalities. The introduction of PET/ computed tomography (CT) in the late 1990s helped clinicians to couple molecular information with anatomic information. Fluorodeoxyglucose (FDG) is an analogue of glucose with a missing hydroxyl group at the 2′ position, which is substituted with positron-emitting fluorine 18, the most widely used radiotracer for PET imaging. FDG-PET/CT imaging enables clinicians to assess cancer biology and perform staging, restaging, and treatment monitoring of cancers.

However, the interpretation of FDG-PET/CT studies is challenging because of the complex physiologic variants, and unusual patterns of FDG uptake. Because FDG is not a tumor-specific tracer, it can accumulate in a variety of benign processes, including benign tumors, and inflammatory, posttraumatic, and iatrogenic conditions. In addition, there is physiologic uptake of FDG in brain, brown fat, muscles, heart, liver, and the genitourinary system. Thus, to overcome these challenges, different special techniques have been introduced in PET/CT imaging. The use of different dynamic maneuvers such as puffed check or open mouth view allows better delineation of tumor margin in head and neck carcinoma. PET/CT enteroclysis is gaining popularity in imaging of the small and large bowels. Efficacy of diuretic FDG-PET/CT studies in the evaluation of genitourinary malignancies is well established in the literature. Dual-time-point imaging (DTPI) and delayed-time-point FDG-PET/CT imaging help in differentiating between malignancy and inflammatory conditions. The use of contrast media during the CT portion helps in better characterization and delineation of the lesion. Metabolic biopsy using FDG-PET/CT yields better results compared with the conventional imaging-guided biopsy. This issue of *PET Clinics* has been prepared in the hope that it will help in the understanding of different special techniques and technical advances in PET/CT imaging, which can help to overcome the diagnostic challenges, resulting in better patient management.

Drs Hanna, Jones, and Chauhan described an overview of conventional imaging-based intervention in clinical practice. With better availability and improving technology, image-guided interventions are increasing in popularity and frequency. Imaging-guided interventions and biopsy and tumor ablations have become key tools in the oncologic practice. Radiologists performing the procedures should be aware of choosing appropriate imaging modality, appropriate instrumentation and techniques, and complications associated with it. PET/CT imaging can help identify the areas of metabolically active

PET Clin 11 (2016) xi–xiii
http://dx.doi.org/10.1016/j.cpet.2015.10.006
1556-8598/16/$ – see front matter © 2016 Published by Elsevier Inc.

pet.theclinics.com

tumor, which can then be specifically targeted for the purpose of biopsy, which would result in a better diagnostic yield.

Drs Kumar, Mukherjee, and Mittal mentioned special techniques in PET/CT imaging for the evaluation of head and neck cancer. FDG-PET/CT plays a significant role in the management of patients with head and neck carcinoma. However, the interpretation of FDG-PET/CT studies in the head and neck is challenging because of the inherently complex anatomy and unusual patterns of FDG uptake after radiation therapy and surgery. In addition, there is physiologic uptake of FDG uptake in brown fat, muscles, vocal cords, and lymphatic system in the head and neck region. In such cases, the use of different dynamic maneuvers, like open-mouth and puffed-cheek techniques, and pharmacologic interventions, such as propranolol and diazepam, may provide useful information about the lesion.

Drs Das, Manchanda, Panda, Sharma, and Gupta shared their experience with a review of literature about recent advances in imaging of small and large bowel using various imaging techniques. The diagnosis of bowel abnormality is challenging in view of the nonspecific clinical presentation. Cross-sectional imaging plays a pivotal role in the evaluation of small and large bowel. With the introduction of hybrid PET/CT and PET/MR imaging scanners combining the advantage of anatomic and functional techniques, there has been a paradigm shift in the imaging of various bowel pathologic abnormalities. Advents of new techniques such as PET/CT enterography and PET/CT colonography bowel imaging have reached a new zenith.

Drs Agarwal, Roy, and Kumar described the role of diuretic 18F-FDG-PET/CT in evaluation of genitourinary malignancies. The interpretation of FDG-PET/CT is often challenging for pelvic pathologies because of the physiologic bowel and urinary tract activity. Intense radiotracer activity in the urinary tract interferes with image interpretation and leads to false negative results in diagnosis and detection of local recurrence and regional lymph node metastases. It is imperative to minimize unnecessary urinary bladder activity to improve the diagnostic yield of PET/CT. Delayed images after forced diuresis with oral hydration give excellent image resolution and have the advantage of imaging the distended bladder with high lesion-to-background contrast.

Drs Higuchi, Suzuki, and Gotoh evaluated the role of PET/CT in radiofrequency ablation (RFA) for malignant pulmonary tumors. Microwave ablation and RFA are local ablative procedures in which thermal, or heat, energy is used and tissues are destroyed by thermocoagulation. RFA is a promising alternative to both surgery and radiotherapy for tumor elimination in patients with primary or metastatic lung malignancy. FDG-PET/CT plays an important role by assessing treatment response and detecting recurrences earlier than conventional imaging. Assessing treatment response also helps in prognostication following RFA.

Drs Cerci, Tabacchi, and Bogoni shared their experience in metabolic biopsy using PET/CT guidance. PET/CT-guided biopsy offers a feasible new approach of potential value in optimizing the diagnostic yield of biopsies. PET/CT-guided biopsy is especially indicated in patients with only a metabolic lesion but no anatomic correspondent lesion and where there is associated necrosis. PET/CT imaging can help identify the areas of metabolically active tumor, which can then be specifically targeted, which would result in better diagnostic yield. PET/CT-guided biopsy might be performed in oncologic patients with metastatic disease in whom tumor transformation/mutation is suspected and in patients with new multiple lesions not known to have malignancy or who has had a prolonged remission or more than one primary malignancy.

Drs Houshmand, Salavati, Segtnan, Grupe, HØilund-Carlsen, and Alavi group, who pioneered in DTPI, described DTPI and delayed-time-point FDG-PET/CT imaging in various clinical settings. FDG is not a tumor-specific tracer; it can accumulate in a variety of benign processes, including benign tumors, and inflammatory, posttraumatic, and iatrogenic conditions. To improve the specificity of FDG for differentiation of malignant and benign lesions, DTPI and delayed-time-point imaging techniques have been introduced. In DTPI and delayed-time-point imaging, the acquisition of the PET studies is done at one standard time point and repeated after a certain amount of time. In addition, the decrease in the background activity in delayed-time points leads to enhanced lesion detection. DTPI has been shown to be useful in both malignant and nonmalignant diseases, such as in the prognostication of patients with lung cancer, diagnosis of primary breast cancer, and detection of atherosclerotic plaques.

Drs Dhull, Rana, and Nazar described the role of various contrast media being used in PET/CT imaging. Contrast agents, also called contrast materials or contrast media, are now an integral part of the diagnostic radiology. State-of-the-art diagnostic PET/CT scan with intravenous or oral contrast gives excellent anatomic details as well as information on tumor vascularization and reduces the need for additional contrast-enhanced diagnostic imaging modalities. Contrast agents (especially positive oral contrast agents) in PET/CT may lead to overestimation of PET attenuation factors. However, this increase/overestimation of standardized uptake value is clinically insignificant.

Rakesh Kumar, MD, PhD
Diagnostic Nuclear Medicine Division
Department of Nuclear Medicine
All India Institute of Medical Sciences
New Delhi 110029, India

E-mail address:
rkphulia@yahoo.com

Overview of Conventional Imaging-based Intervention in Clinical Practice

Ramez Hanna, MD, Lisa P. Jones, MD, PhD,
Anil Chauhan, MD*

KEYWORDS

- Image guided • Interventions • Biopsy • Ablation • Tumor • CT • Ultrasonography

KEY POINTS

- With better availability and improving technology, image-guided interventions are increasingly being performed.
- Ultrasonography-guided and/or computed tomography (CT)–guided biopsy and tumor ablations are the most commonly performed oncologic procedures using imaging guidance.
- Radiologists performing the procedures should not only be aware of risks associated with the interventions but also the various maneuvers to minimize those risks.
- PET-CT imaging can help identify the areas of metabolically active tumor (in the presence of necrosis, or in patients with history of prior treatment), which can then be specifically targeted for the purpose of biopsy under imaging guidance.

INTRODUCTION

In this evolving era of individualized oncologic medicine, image-guided interventions are increasing in popularity and frequency for several reasons, including (1) technical improvements that have led to increased efficacy and safety; (2) preference for minimally invasive techniques rather than surgical options; and (3) an increase in the number of situations in which tissue diagnosis is required, such as for clinical trials or biological/molecular tumor profiling for targeted therapy.[1–8] The most common imaging-guided interventions are biopsy and tumor ablation, which are commonly performed across the nation and have become key tools in the armamentarium of oncologic practices for the diagnosis and treatment of disease.[1–8]

This article discusses the indications, contraindications, techniques, and various considerations for some of the most commonly performed image-guided interventions, namely conventional imaging-guided biopsies and tumor ablation. It also briefly addresses the role of PET imaging and future imaging techniques in the context of these biopsies, which are addressed in other articles in this issue.

GENERAL CONSIDERATIONS
The Importance of Guidance

One of the primary advantages of image guidance is a decrease in both the nondiagnostic rate and in the number of complications. For example, in a study by Maya and colleagues[9] of random native kidney biopsies, none of the image-guided biopsies were nondiagnostic compared with 16% in the nonguided group. In addition, the rate of significant hemorrhage was significantly reduced,

The authors have nothing to disclose.
Division of Abdominal Imaging, Department of Radiology, University of Pennsylvania, 3400 Spruce Street, Philadelphia, PA 19104, USA
* Corresponding author.
E-mail address: Anil.Chauhan@uphs.upenn.edu

PET Clin 11 (2016) 1–12
http://dx.doi.org/10.1016/j.cpet.2015.07.004

with none of the image-guided cohort requiring transfusion, compared with 11% of the nonguided group.

Choosing the Imaging Modality

Invariably, ultrasonography is the mainstay tool for image guidance of biopsies.[7,10] The mantra "If it can be seen it can be done" applies to ultrasonography as a guiding modality in most scenarios. Ultrasonography machines are portable and readily available in most radiology centers. In addition, the ultrasonography probes are easy to handle and allow real-time visualization of the needle and the target lesion. Color Doppler imaging also plays an important role during interventions to evaluate for vascular structures in the path of the needle and to assess the vascularity of the target lesion. Other advantages include the lack of ionizing radiation and real-time evaluation for potential postbiopsy complications such as arteriovenous fistulas and hemorrhage. Complications such as hemorrhage (if detected on postbiopsy scan) can usually be managed effectively with pressure application, while the patient is still on the biopsy table.

Despite its advantages, there are situations in which visualization of the target lesion may be suboptimal by ultrasonography, either because of patient-related factors, such as high body mass index, small sonographic windows caused by bowel gas, or because of small size and/or deep location of the target lesion. In these situations, computed tomography (CT) guidance may be preferred.[11]

Magnetic resonance (MR) imaging is a newer entrant to imaging guidance, and has been primarily used in breast and prostate biopsies.[12,13] It is yet not widely available, and is an expensive modality compared with ultrasonography and CT examinations. However, techniques such as MR imaging/transrectal ultrasonography fusion for prostate biopsies are becoming increasing popular because they combine the excellent tissue contrast of MR imaging with the real-time guidance capability of ultrasonography.[14]

Instrumentation and Technique

Image-guided biopsies are performed with a variety of different sized needles, which tend to be smaller (25–20 G) for fine-needle aspiration biopsies (FNABs), and larger (20–11 G) for core biopsies (**Table 1**). Core biopsies have the advantage of providing a greater amount of cellular material for analysis, and also allow the cellular architecture of the tumor to be examined, which may be critical in the diagnosis of lymphoma and certain sarcomas.[15–17] In addition, the greater amount of material obtained by core biopsy

Table 1	
Commonly used needle sizes and their use in imaging-guided biopsies	
Needle Size	**Common Indications/Comments**
27 G FNAB	Thyroid nodules, lidocaine injection
25 G FNAB	Soft tissue masses/lymph nodes
22 G FNAB	Deeper soft tissue masses/lymph nodes, solid organs
20 G FNAB	Deeper soft tissue masses/lymph nodes, solid organs (needle more visible through subcutaneous fat on ultrasound)
20 G core	Used occasionally in high-risk patients
18 G core	Most commonly used core biopsy needle
16 G core	Random organ biopsies, soft tissue sarcoma (16 G preferred)

permits additional molecular testing, as may be necessary in both clinical and research settings.[15,16] In core biopsies, although larger needles have the theoretic advantage of higher diagnostic yield, this is countered by the higher potential risk of bleeding and organ injury. Radiologists performing the procedure, while collaborating with the pathologist and the requesting physician, should judiciously weigh the risk against the benefit of one technique compared with another.

Fine-needle aspiration biopsy

FNABs are often used in the following situations: (1) suspected metastatic deposit in a patient with known primary malignancy, when only a limited number of cells are required to establish a diagnosis; (2) small lesions, for which core biopsy may be risky or difficult (eg, thyroid nodules); and (3) to confirm areas of viable tumor in the setting of complex cystic or necrotic lesions (before core biopsy). In FNAB, a thin needle is introduced into the lesion under imaging guidance, and is moved in a to-and-fro manner, resulting in collection of cells via a capillary-action mechanism (**Fig. 1**). At our institution, cytopathologists are available on site to assess a portion of the specimen for adequacy and to determine whether a core biopsy is necessary. Any portion of the specimen that is not examined on site is submitted to the cytopathology department in solution for additional analysis or flow cytometry as required.[18]

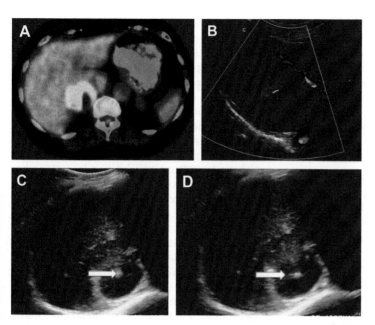

Fig. 1. PET-CT examination in a 79-year-old female patient with history of uterine carcinosarcoma shows right adrenal lesion (A). Because there is a focal area of necrosis along the medial aspect, and there was a small risk of pneumothorax with a posterior approach, it was decided to take a transhepatic approach. Ultrasonography examination confirmed the presence of right adrenal lesion (B). Fine-needle aspiration was performed, noting proximal (C) and distal (D) positions of the needle as a part of to-and-fro motions (arrows).

Core biopsy

There are several core needle biopsy systems available for clinical use, including manual and automated systems offered in a variety of needle gauges and specimen lengths. To obtain a core, these devices use 2 different intercalated needles: an inner, smaller needle that collects the sample; and an outer, larger needle that cuts the sample defined by the inner needle. In some systems, the inner needle is deployed and positioned into the target before the outer cutting needle is deployed, allowing the exact site of the core to be visualized before the sample is acquired (Fig. 2). This type of system is preferred when precise positioning is required; for example, when the target is close to a critical structure or is very small. In other systems, the needle fires a certain distance forward into the tissues at the

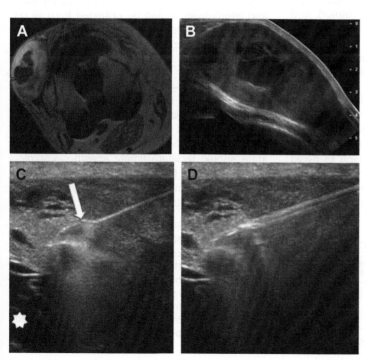

Fig. 2. MR imaging examination in a 61-year-old male patient shows a large subcutaneous mass at the level of the right knee (A). Ultrasonography examination confirms the presence of large mass with central necrotic region (B). Ultrasonography-guided core biopsy is shown here with full stretch of the inner needle (C), noting the beveled notch (arrow; the distal margin of the tissue to be biopsied). (D) The outer needle deployed to the beveled notch, at which point the needle is withdrawn to collect the sample. Note that the area of central necrosis (star) was avoided.

time of sampling, and therefore the radiologist must anticipate the track and length of the outer needle, to avoid less precise sampling (**Fig. 3**). In this system, the needle tip should be placed just inside the proximal aspect of the lesion. The advantage of this system is that the core is circular in cross section (as opposed to semicircular in the other system) and theoretically more tissue is acquired.

Coaxial system

Another important consideration is the use of a coaxial technique, especially for the solid organs. Hatfield and colleagues[19] in a study of 1060 consecutive patients undergoing liver and renal biopsies, showed that the use of the co-axial technique resulted in slightly fewer overall complications (2.6% vs 3.4%). However, these results were not statistically significant. In general, the coaxial technique offers a safe pathway for lesions in difficult locations, especially when multiple samples are required. At our institution, we typically use the coaxial technique for CT-guided biopsies, in which positioning is often difficult and time consuming. However, we generally do not use the coaxial technique for ultrasonography, for which real-time imaging generally permits rapid and reproducible positioning of a needle into the target.

Technical Maneuvers

A variety of techniques and maneuvers have been described to aid in lesion visualization and access, and to improve patient and operator comfort, and the commonly encountered scenarios are briefly described here.

First, patient and operator comfort can significantly reduce the difficultly of a challenging biopsy. Unless specified differently later, the supine position is the most comfortable position for patients.[7] It reduces patient anxiety and allows for prolonged breath holds for biopsies near the diaphragm. Ideally, most liver biopsies should be performed using a subcostal approach to avoid the risk of pneumothorax or injuring intercostal neurovascular bundles. In certain instances (liver-dome lesions, high-riding liver, and subcapsular lateral right hepatic lobe lesions), an intercostal approach may be preferred. In the intercostal approach, it is crucial to place the needle just above the superior margin of the rib to avoid the neurovascular bundle, which lies along the inferior margin of the rib.[5,6,20]

When a lesion is adjacent to a critical organ, hydrodisplacement can be used to create separation between the target lesion and the critical structure. In this technique, sterile water, saline, dextrose, or gas (only for CT) may be infused in a plane between the two structures.[20] Another technique is to displace the organ (usually bowel) from the target path using pressure with the ultrasonography transducer. In some cases, a transorgan approach is the best choice. In particular, right adrenal mass or anterolateral right superior kidney mass may at times be best approached by a trans-hepatic approach (see **Fig. 1**). Less conventional routes, such as the transvaginal and transrectal approaches, should be considered for pelvic cases that are not readily accessible by the percutaneous route.

In addition, it should be emphasized that needle penetration of most solid abdominal organs should be performed during patient breath holding to avoid the theoretic risk of causing shear injury to organ capsules and to reduce the risk of hemorrhage.[20–23]

PATIENT PREPARATION

A written consent explaining the procedure, risks, and alternatives should be obtained from all patients, or from a designated representative, before performing the procedure.

Fasting

When moderate sedation is planned or before deep visceral biopsies, the patient should be fasting for at least 6 hours. Should a major complication occur, having the patient in the fasting state should facilitate timely anesthesia/surgical intervention.[23,24] For superficial biopsies such as thyroid and subcutaneous nodules/lymph nodes, fasting is not required.

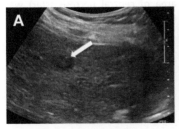 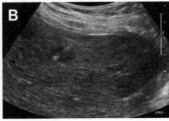

Fig. 3. Ultrasonography shows a core-biopsy needle system, in which the needle tip (*arrow*) before the biopsy is positioned just inside the lesion (*A*), and the outer needle moves forward up to a predetermined length (*B*) to receive the sample (in this case 1.3 cm).

Preprocedural Laboratory Evaluation

Before deep visceral biopsies, a complete blood count and International Normalized Ratio (INR) should be performed to determine the patient's baseline hematocrit and to evaluate the patient's coagulation status. An INR of 1.5 is generally used as an upper limit for solid abdominal organ biopsy, and a platelet count of 50,000 per µL is typically used as a minimum for platelet count.[25,26]

Medications

As part of the preprocedure evaluation, the medications should be reviewed to assess whether the patient is taking the anticoagulant and/or antiplatelet medications. For certain types of biopsies, it may be prudent to temporarily hold such medications before the biopsy to minimize bleeding complications. However, it may be worthwhile to consult with the referring physician before altering the medications, to determine the potential risk to the patient. Note that the exact duration that an anticoagulant/antiplatelet agent must be held before biopsy depends both on the type of biopsy and the medication. **Table 2** details guidelines on anticoagulation/antiplatelet medications adopted at our institute.

Table 2
The guidelines regarding common anticoagulation/antiplatelet medications at our institute

Medication	Preprocedure	Postprocedure
Aspirin	5 d, if possible	Restart at 24–48 h
NSAIDs	Do not stop	Avoid for 48 h
Clopidogrel	5 d prior	Restart at 24–48 h
Coumadin	3–5 d prior; normalized INR 1.5. In consultation with PCP	Restart after procedure
Heparin	6 h prior	Restart at 6–12 h
LMWH	6–12 h prior	Restart at 12–24 h
Rivaroxaban	24–48 h prior (longer with renal failure)	Restart at 24–48 h

Abbreviations: LMWH, low-molecular-weight heparin; NSAIDs, nonsteroidal antiinflammatory drugs; PCP, primary care provider.

Time-out

Part of standard practice now is the use of the preprocedural time-out (Universal Protocol by the Joint Commission on Accreditation of Healthcare Organizations), which has been widely adopted and has significantly reduced the risk of wrong-sided procedures and avoidable complications.[27]

Pain Control

Most, if not all, biopsies are performed under local anesthetics. Typically, 1% lidocaine with or without epinephrine is administered to the skin surface and subcutaneous fat.[4,7] For deep procedures, lidocaine is also administered to the region of the organ capsule, because this is often the most sensitive area. In some cases, an anxiolytic medication such as intravenous lorazepam (Ativan) may also be helpful as minimal sedation. Usually, adequate pain control can be obtained in this manner. In moderate sedation (conscious sedation), the combination of intravenous fentanyl citrate 25 to 100 µg and intravenous midazolam hydrochloride (Versed) 1 to 2 mg is commonly used to achieve appropriate sedation. Conscious sedation should be performed according to hospital/clinic policies, with appropriate monitoring by a nurse during the procedure.[24,28,29]

Postprocedural Care

For superficial biopsies, patients are discharged home immediately postprocedure, assuming no complication is identified on the postbiopsy imaging. For solid organ biopsies, patients are monitored by radiology nursing for 2 hours, because major hemorrhage typically manifests clinically 2 to 4 hours following biopsy.[5] If the patient develops symptoms or signs of major hemorrhage (worsening pain, dizziness, hypotension, tachycardia, and so forth) during the period of observation, repeat ultrasonography or CT examination may be performed, with additional interventions as necessary depending on the imaging findings and the patient's clinical status. Any patient who is being considered for a moderate sedation must be accompanied by an individual who will be responsible for the patient (including transportation home) after the patient is discharged.

Some of the more commonly performed image-guided biopsies are addressed in more detail later.

LIVER

Ultrasonography is the modality of choice in biopsying the liver lesions that can be visualized (see **Fig. 3**). Initial imaging is performed with both grayscale and color Doppler to identify the targets and to map bile ducts, major vessels, and other anatomic structures that should be avoided. In addition, target vascularity is evaluated to maximize the probability of sampling a viable region. It is preferable to traverse normal liver before entry of the target, because of the theoretic increased risk of hemorrhage if the subcapsular aspect of a lesion traversed. As another consideration, when multiple hepatic lesions are present, the best visualized and least risky lesion should be selected as the target.[6]

In patients with cirrhosis, there are several additional important considerations. First, if moderate ascites is present, the liver may become mobile, such that targeting a specific small lesion becomes challenging, if not impossible. Placing the patient in the left lateral decubitus position may shift the fluid away from the liver. However, if extensive ascites is present, a paracentesis may be necessary before the biopsy.[7,30] Another common issue is coagulopathy related to the hepatic insufficiency. Therefore, in this patient population it is critical to assess for coagulopathy so that fresh frozen plasma and other interventions can be considered before proceeding with the biopsy.[31,32] In addition, the presence of portosystemic shunts can lead to significant bleeding should they be traversed. Prior imaging should be reviewed to determine the location of such shunts.

The diagnostic yield for targeted liver biopsy is excellent, ranging from 79% to 99%, including lesions less than 1 cm.[22,33,34] In addition, the complication rate is low. In a study by Giorgio and colleagues[35] of 16,628 patients who had ultrasonography-guided liver biopsies, no deaths or major hemorrhagic episodes were reported. In 0.3% of patients, mild hemoperitoneum was detected. Pain is the most common minor complication and was likely related to stretching of the liver capsule and/or peritoneal irritation from a small amount of hemorrhage. In a minority of cases, the pain may be referred to the left shoulder because of diaphragmatic irritation. The incidence of pain was reported as 9.3% of 715 cases in the study by Weigand and Weigand.[34]

KIDNEYS

In the past, the standard of care was to resect any enhancing mass that could not be characterized as an angiomyolipoma, and therefore there was little role for biopsy. However, several factors have led to increasing interest in renal mass sampling, including (1) improved sensitivity and specificity of percutaneous biopsy, (2) increase in the number of incidentally detected renal masses, and (3) the requirement to characterize a renal lesion before percutaneous ablation.[2,36]

Renal biopsies have a reported sensitivity of 70% to 100% and specificity of 100% for focal masses.[7,36] However, note that the size and nature of the lesion is an important determinant of success. For example, Rybicki and colleagues[37] (2003) showed that the overall sensitivity and negative predictive value for renal biopsies are 97% and 89% respectively for lesions measuring 4 to 6 cm (this included both cystic and solid lesions). When subgroup analysis for cystic lesions was performed, the sensitivity and negative predictive value significantly decreased to 33% and 87%.

The kidney is a highly perfused organ and therefore attention to the coagulation parameters is important. In addition, it should be noted that in uremic patients the platelets may be dysfunctional and therefore clotting may not be as effective.[36] For ultrasonography guidance, patients are usually placed in the prone or contralateral decubitus positions. For CT guidance, the prone position is preferred to the decubitus position, because this position decreases the risk of traversing the pleural space and generally allows better visualization of the kidneys. The main disadvantage of the prone position is that anterolateral exophytic lesions may be difficult to visualize, especially by ultrasonography.[36]

Hemorrhage is the most commonly reported complication, and primarily occurs into 3 locations (1) the collecting system, resulting in hematuria (associated with traversing the renal medulla); (2) subcapsular space; and (3) perinephric space.[36] Hemorrhage is reported in as many as 91% of cases; however, severe hemorrhage is rare, with only 1% of cases requiring a transfusion, and 0.1% of patients require nephrectomy.[38] Infection is exceedingly rare. However, biopsies should be delayed in patients with an active urinary tract infection to minimize the risk. Pneumothorax is also rare, and, as previously mentioned, the risk may be minimized with attention to patient positioning and visualization of the pleural space. Other complications include arteriovenous fistula and pseudoaneurysm. These complications can sometimes be detected on the postprocedure Doppler evaluation of the biopsy site. In addition, there is a theoretic risk of tumor seeding. However, according to Uppot and colleagues[36] there have been only 7 reported cases of tumor seeding with renal biopsy. Therefore, the risk is very low, and likely has decreased further with improvements in technique.

SPLEEN

The spleen is a highly vascularized organ and therefore splenic biopsies are rarely performed because of the perceived increased risk of hemorrhage.[6,23,28] However, indications for splenic biopsy are uncommon. The typical indication for splenic biopsy is an indeterminate solid or cystic lesion that would change the management of patient; for example, a lesion in a patient with a known history of malignancy and no other potential sites of metastasis, or an enlarging splenic lesion that is suspected to be malignant.[3,10] In a 10-year retrospective review by Lucey and colleagues,[39] the investigators performed 24 biopsies in 23 patients. The most common indication for the biopsy was known primary malignancy with a splenic lesion. Lymphoma was the most common malignancy.

In a meta-analysis by McInnes and colleagues[3] the investigators were able to show that, based on 4 high- quality studies (including 639 patients), the sensitivity of splenic biopsies was 87% and the specificity was 96.4%. The major complication rate was 2.2%, which included hemorrhage and pneumothorax. The complications related to hemorrhage were treated with transfusions or rarely splenectomy. The most common minor complication from the procedure was pain. The complication rates were slightly higher for core needle biopsies (5.8%) versus fine-needle aspiration (4.3%).

OMENTAL/MESENTERIC/RETROPERITONEAL MASSES

Peritoneal carcinomatosis-related deposits are the most commonly biopsied omental/mesenteric lesions. Although carcinomatosis can be confidently identified on cross-sectional imaging, biopsy may be required to obtain tissue for diagnosis or molecular testing for targeted chemotherapy. Other common indications for mesenteric/peritoneal biopsy include other mesenteric masses such as carcinoid tumor, desmoid tumors, fibrous sclerosing mesenteritis, and adenopathy.[4,7,40]

Ultrasonography is often the modality of choice because it permits real-time evaluation of the bowel or blood vessels, and transducer pressure may be applied to displace segments of bowel. In the retroperitoneum, CT is usually the preferred imaging modality, particularly if the lymph nodes are small or deep (**Fig. 4**). It should be emphasized that colonic injury is associated with a greater risk for infection and abscess formation, compared with small bowel injury. Therefore, although small bowel loops may sometimes be traversed safely with a small-gauge needle, the colon should be avoided. In cases in which a safe percutaneous biopsy is not possible, the transgastric or transduodenal approaches offered by gastroenterologists may be options.

The reported yield from biopsy of omental/mesenteric masses is less than from biopsy of the solid organs, with the success rate ranging between 77% and 89%.[7] The success rate may be even lower following chemotherapy, because of heterogeneity related to showing treatment-related fibrotic changes, which may lead to sampling error.

PELVIC NODES

The biopsy of enlarged pelvic lymph nodes is commonly requested in patients with history of primary genitourinary or gastrointestinal malignancies. CT is the imaging modality of choice. For internal iliac chain nodes, a transgluteal approach is commonly used, with the needle track traversing along the lateral edge of the sacrum and along the caudal part of sciatic notch, to avoid injury to the sacral neural plexus (**Fig. 5**).

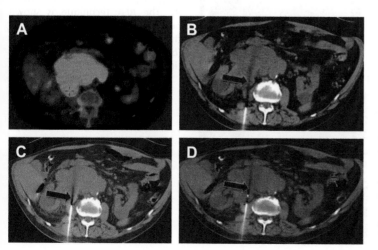

Fig. 4. PET-CT examination in an 80-year-old female patient shows fluorodeoxyglucose-avid mass in the retroperitoneum (*A*). The CT-guided core-biopsy technique is shown here, noting the coaxial needle positioned halfway through the lesion of interest (*B*), followed by the needle tip at the edge of the lesion (*C*), and then the cutting biopsy needle being advanced (*D*). Note the beam-hardening artifact from the needle (*black arrows*), which can be used to anticipate the needle path.

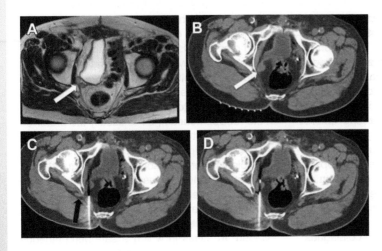

Fig. 5. MR imaging examination in a 62-year-old male patient with a history of bladder cancer shows enlarged right obturator lymph nodes (*white arrows*; *A*, *B*), confirmed on prebiopsy CT examination (*B*). (*C*) The coaxial needle being advanced to the posterior margin of the target lesion, noting that the passage is along the lateral margin of the sacrum to avoid the sciatic nerve plexus located along the lateral aspect (*black arrow*). (*D*) The lesion being biopsied.

Anterior and anterolateral approaches are typically used for external iliac and inguinal nodes. Ultrasonography is the modality of choice, but CT is preferred for more deeply positioned lymph nodes.

TUMOR ABLATION

The imaging-guided ablative procedures are discussed here. Ideally, an ablative procedure should be able to produce a 5-mm to 10-mm tumor-free margin, and be performed on a lesion that is targetable without adding significant risk.[41,42] There are several methods available for tumor ablation, including radiofrequency ablation (RFA), cryoablation (CA), microwave ablation, and ethanol ablation. RFA and CA, the two most commonly performed ablations, are the focus here.

Radiofrequency Ablation

RFA has gained significant popularity in recent years as a safe and effective alternative for management of lesions in patients who would otherwise be considered terminal.

In RFA, a probe is placed in the center of the lesion under imaging guidance and prongs are deployed to create a treatment area of dimensions that vary according to the specific device selected (**Fig. 6**). Lesions are treated (burned) through tissue heating generated from frictional

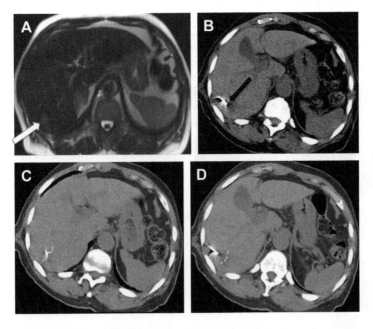

Fig. 6. MR imaging examination in a 79-year-old patient with a history of clear cell renal cell carcinoma shows a metastatic lesion in the right hepatic lobe (*white arrow*; *A*). The RFA technique is shown here, with the RFA needle tip at the proximal margin of the lesion (*black arrow*; *B*). (*C*, *D*) Multiple tines deployed.

forces related to alternating electrical current in the radiofrequency range (375–480 kHz).[41,42] The heat from the radiofrequency probe dissipates into the surrounding soft tissues through thermal diffusion, which causes coagulative necrosis of the target tissue. As the distance from probe increases, there is a significant decline of temperature, avoiding surrounding tissue injury.[43]

One of the major limitations of using RFA is the heterogeneity of energy deposition, also known as the heat-sink effect. This effect occurs in the vicinity of large (>3 mm) blood vessels, and is caused by heat dissipation into adjacent flowing blood. This dissipation produces a local reduction in the temperature, which may decrease to less than that necessary to produce coagulative necrosis.

In the abdomen, RFA is most commonly used to treat hepatic and renal lesions. In the liver, two of the most common indications are ablation of hepatocellular carcinomas (HCC) to control disease while awaiting transplantation and the treatment of metastases. RFA has been shown to be effective in HCCs less than 3 cm. In lesions greater than 3 cm a combination of therapies (including transarterial chemoembolization) with or without RFA may be more effective than RFA alone.[44] In a systemic review by Sutherland and colleagues,[45] RFA of the HCCs was deemed to be safe and more effective compared with other therapies, including percutaneous transarterial injection and transarterial chemoembolization. With respect to the utility of RFA in the setting of colorectal metastatic disease, the results are not as promising. However, a recent report by Solbitati and colleagues[46] with a minimum 3-year follow-up of 99 consecutive patients with 202 hepatic metastases revealed that RFA is noninferior to surgical resection. Furthermore, RFA may have a role in a combined approach to hepatic metastases in which a partial hepatectomy is performed followed by intraoperative ultrasonography-guided RFA of any residual lesions.

For renal lesions, the primary indication for RFA is for treatment of renal cell carcinoma in patients with comorbidities precluding surgical intervention.[47] A biopsy of the lesion is typically obtained before ablation treatment. Injury to the colon, adrenal gland, and ureter are additional risks that can sometimes be ameliorated through techniques such as hydrodisplacement and ureteral stent placement.[47] Success of the procedure depends on the size, location, and histology of the lesion.[47,48]

Cryoablation

Cryoablation (CA) is an alternative to RFA for percutaneous treatment of malignant lesions. It operates by a different mechanism. CA destroys the tumor cells by creating a cooling cytotoxic temperature as low as -160°C.[44] A significant advantage of CA is the high visibility of the ice ball (indicating the treated area) on imaging (commonly CT) created during cryoablation (**Fig. 7**). As with RFA, the probe is placed in the center of the tumor under ultrasonography or CT guidance.[41,42,49] A 5-mm ablation margin beyond the tumor should be considered sufficient, but many operators prefer a margin of 10 mm if feasible, because the ill-defined tumor, perilesional hemorrhage, and the needle artifact can make margin assessment difficult. Healing tends to be faster in CA compared with RFA.

CA is increasingly being used in treatment of renal tumors and bone lesions. CA has greater overall bleeding risk compared with RFA, and also tends to cause delayed bleeding as a complication.[44] Therefore, many investigators

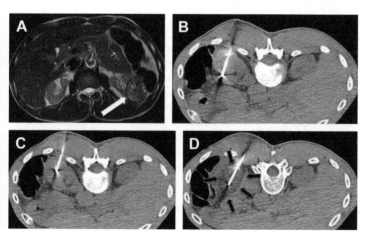

Fig. 7. MR imaging examination in a 59-year-old male patient shows a 4.8-cm mass (*white arrow*; *A*). (*B*, *C*) The cryoablation technique is shown, with 2 separate needles (total of 3 needles were used in this large lesion). (*D*) An ice ball (*black arrows*) has been created surrounding the needle as a result of cryoablation.

recommend delaying anticoagulation for 2 weeks after the procedure. Overall success rate of CA in renal tumors is up to 97%, with a complication rate of up to 7%.[41,42]

Role of PET–Computed Tomography

The role of PET/CT scan fusion for guiding biopsies is discussed here. As discussed by Kobayashi and colleagues,[1] PET-CT scans can offer important ancillary information that can increase the diagnostic yield for biopsies. Specifically in the setting of a large, partially necrotic lesion, PET-CT is able to show which parts of the lesion are metabolically active and should be targeted for biopsy. In addition, in the setting of multiple lesions, PET-CT can show which lesions are most metabolically active and therefore offer the highest diagnostic yield from biopsies. In addition, in the setting of distorted anatomy related to postsurgical change/radiation change, PET-CT can show discrete nodules or areas of suspected malignancy that would be occult on conventional imaging. In a study by Cerci and colleagues,[50] 130 biopsies were performed under PET/CT guidance with a diagnostic yield of 98.5%.

With future advances in fusion imaging, PET/CT and ultrasonography fusion will offer additional advantages for diagnostic biopsies and further improvement in their yield. Other technologies, such as electromagnetic tracking with PET/CT and ultrasonography fusion, will continue to improve the utility of percutaneous biopsies.[51]

SUMMARY

This article discusses some of the technical considerations for image-guided biopsies. It also focuses on site-specific biopsies, such as liver, spleen, renal, and soft tissue biopsies, in the abdomen with special focus on indeterminate lesions. It also briefly discusses the emerging role of PET imaging and other technologies that will further improve the diagnostic yield of image-guided biopsies.

REFERENCES

1. Kobayashi K, Bhargava P, Raja S, et al. Image-guided biopsy: what the interventional radiologist needs to know about PET/CT. RadioGraphics 2012;32(5):1483–501.
2. Beland MD, Mayo-Smith WW, Dupuy DE, et al. Diagnostic yield of 58 consecutive imaging-guided biopsies of solid renal masses: should we biopsy all that are indeterminate? AJR Am J Roentgenol 2007;188(3):792–7.
3. McInnes MDF, Kielar AZ, Macdonald DB. Percutaneous image-guided biopsy of the spleen: systematic review and meta-analysis of the complication rate and diagnostic accuracy. Radiology 2011; 260(3):699–708.
4. Spencer JA, Weston MJ, Saidi SA, et al. Clinical utility of image-guided peritoneal and omental biopsy. Nat Rev Clin Oncol 2010;7(11):623–31.
5. Rockey DC, Caldwell SH, Goodman ZD, et al. Liver biopsy. Hepatology 2008;49(3):1017–44.
6. Winter TC, Lee FT, Hinshaw JL. Ultrasound-guided biopsies in the abdomen and pelvis. Ultrasound Q 2008;24(1):45–68.
7. Khati NJ, Gorodenker J, Hill MC. Ultrasound-guided biopsies of the abdomen. Ultrasound Q 2011;27(4): 255–68.
8. Berland LL, Silverman SG, Gore RM, et al. Managing incidental findings on abdominal CT: white paper of the ACR incidental findings committee. J Am Coll Radiol 2010;7(10):754–73.
9. Maya ID, Maddela P, Barker J, et al. Percutaneous renal biopsy: comparison of blind and real-time ultrasound-guided technique. Semin Dial 2007;20(4): 355–8.
10. Singh AK, Shankar S, Gervais DA, et al. Image-guided percutaneous splenic interventions. RadioGraphics 2012;32(2):523–34.
11. Gupta S, Nguyen HL, Morello FA Jr, et al. Various approaches for CT-guided percutaneous biopsy of deep pelvic lesions: anatomic and technical considerations. RadioGraphics 2004;24(1): 175–89.
12. Peltier A, Aoun F, Lemort M, et al. MRI-targeted biopsies versus systematic transrectal ultrasound guided biopsies for the diagnosis of localized prostate cancer in biopsy naïve men. Biomed Res Int 2015;2015(23):1–6.
13. Imschweiler T, Haueisen H, Kampmann G, et al. MRI-guided vacuum-assisted breast biopsy: comparison with stereotactically guided and ultrasound-guided techniques. Eur Radiol 2013; 24(1):128–35.
14. Sonn GA, Chang E, Natarajan S, et al. Value of targeted prostate biopsy using magnetic resonance–ultrasound fusion in men with prior negative biopsy and elevated prostate-specific antigen. Eur Urol 2014;65(4):809–15.
15. Stewart C, Coldewey J, Stewart IS. Comparison of fine needle aspiration cytology needle core biopsy in the diagnosis of radiologically detected abdominal lesions. J Clin Pathol 2002;55(2):93–7.
16. Amador-Ortiz C, Chen L, Hassan A, et al. Combined core needle biopsy and fine-needle aspiration with ancillary studies correlate highly with traditional techniques in the diagnosis of nodal-based lymphoma. Am J Clin Pathol 2011;135(4): 516–24.

17. Nguyen B, Halpern C, Olimpiadi Y, et al. Core needle biopsy is a safe and accurate initial diagnostic procedure for suspected lymphoma. Am J Surg 2014;208(6):1003–8.

18. Wu M, Burstein DE. Fine needle aspiration. Cancer Invest 2004;22(4):620–8.

19. Hatfield MK, Beres RA, Sane SS, et al. Percutaneous imaging-guided solid organ core needle biopsy: coaxial versus noncoaxial method. AJR Am J Roentgenol 2008;190(2):413–7.

20. Sainani NI, Arellano RS, Shyn PB, et al. The challenging image-guided abdominal mass biopsy: established and emerging techniques "if you can see it, you can biopsy it." Abdom Imaging 2013; 38(4):672–96.

21. Fisher AJ, Paulson EK, Sheafor DH, et al. Small lymph nodes of the abdomen, pelvis, and retroperitoneum: Usefulness of sonographically guided biopsy. Radiology 1997;205(1):185–90.

22. Yu S, Liew CT, Lau WY, et al. US-guided percutaneous biopsy of small (≤1-cm) hepatic lesions. Radiology 2001;218(1):195–9.

23. O'Malley ME, Wood BJ, Boland GW, et al. Percutaneous imaging-guided biopsy of the spleen. AJR 1999;172(3):661–5.

24. Lieberman S, Libson E, Sella T, et al. Percutaneous image-guided splenic procedures: update on indications, technique, complications, and outcomes. Semin Ultrasound CT MR 2007;28(1): 57–63.

25. O'Connor SD, Taylor AJ, Williams EC, et al. Coagulation concepts update. AJR Am J Roentgenol 2009; 193(6):1656–64.

26. Malloy PC, Grassi CJ, Kundu S, et al. Consensus guidelines for periprocedural management of coagulation status and hemostasis risk in percutaneous image-guided interventions. J Vasc Interv Radiol 2009;20(7 Suppl):S240–9.

27. Johnson CD, Krecke KN, Miranda R, et al. Developing a radiology quality and safety program: a primer. RadioGraphics 2009;29(4):951–9.

28. Keogan MT, Freed KS, Paulson EK, et al. Imaging-guided percutaneous biopsy of focal splenic lesions: update on safety and effectiveness. AJR Am J Roentgenol 1999;172(4):933–7.

29. Paulsen SD, Nghiem HV, Negussie E, et al. Evaluation of imaging-guided core biopsy of pancreatic masses. AJR Am J Roentgenol 2006;187(3): 769–72.

30. Grant A, Neuberger J. Guidelines on the use of liver biopsy in clinical practice. British Society of Gastroenterology. Gut 1999;45:IV1–11.

31. Abdel-Wahab OI, Healy B, Dzik WH. Effect of fresh-frozen plasma transfusion on prothrombin time and bleeding in patients with mild coagulation abnormalities. Transfusion 2006;46(8): 1279–85.

32. Youssef W. Role of fresh frozen plasma infusion in correction of coagulopathy of chronic liver disease: a dual phase study. Am J Gastroenterol 2003;98(6): 1391–4.

33. Matsubara J, Okusaka T, Morizane C, et al. Ultrasound-guided percutaneous pancreatic tumor biopsy in pancreatic cancer: a comparison with metastatic liver tumor biopsy, including sensitivity, specificity, and complications. J Gastroenterol 2008;43(3):225–32.

34. Weigand K, Weigand K. Percutaneous liver biopsy: retrospective study over 15 years comparing 287 inpatients with 428 outpatients. J Gastroenterol Hepatol 2009;24(5):792–9.

35. Giorgio A, Tarantino L, de Stefano G, et al. Complications after interventional sonography of focal liver lesions - a 22-year single-center experience. J Ultrasound Med 2003;22(2):193–205.

36. Uppot RN, Harisinghani MG, Gervais DA. Imaging-guided percutaneous renal biopsy: rationale and approach. AJR Am J Roentgenol 2010;194(6): 1443–9.

37. Rybicki FJ, Shu KM, Cibas ES, et al. Percutaneous biopsy of renal masses: sensitivity and negative predictive value stratified by clinical setting and size of masses. AJR Am J Roentgenol 2003; 180(5):1281–7.

38. Walker PD. The renal biopsy. Arch Pathol Lab Med 2009;133(2):181–8.

39. Lucey BC, Boland GW, Maher MM, et al. Percutaneous nonvascular splenic intervention: a 10-year review. AJR 2002;179(6):1591–6.

40. Souza FF, Mortelé KJ, Cibas ES, et al. Predictive value of percutaneous imaging-guided biopsy of peritoneal and omental masses: results in 111 patients. AJR Am J Roentgenol 2009;192(1):131–6.

41. Breen DJ, Lencioni R. Image-guided ablation of primary liver and renal tumours. Nat Rev Clin Oncol 2015;12(3):175–86.

42. Georgiades C, Rodriguez R. Renal tumor ablation. Tech Vasc Interv Radiol 2013;16(4):230–8.

43. Hong K, Georgiades C. Radiofrequency ablation: mechanism of action and devices. J Vasc Interv Radiol 2010;21(S):S179–86.

44. Hinshaw JL, Lubner MG, Ziemlewicz TJ, et al. Percutaneous tumor ablation tools: microwave, radiofrequency, or cryoablation—what should you use and why? Radiographics 2014;34(5): 1344–62.

45. Sutherland LM, Williams JAR, Padbury RTA, et al. Radiofrequency ablation of liver tumors: a systematic review. Arch Surg 2006;141(2):181–90.

46. Solbiati L, Ahmed M, Cova L, et al. Small liver colorectal metastases treated with percutaneous radiofrequency ablation: local response rate and long-term survival with up to 10-year follow-up. Radiology 2012;265(3):958–68.

47. Zagoria RJ. Imaging-guided radiofrequency ablation of renal masses. Radiographics 2004;24(Suppl 1):S59–71.

48. Park JJ, Park BK, Park SY, et al. Percutaneous radiofrequency ablation of sporadic Bosniak III or IV lesions: treatment techniques and short-term outcomes. J Vasc Interv Radiol 2015;26(1):46–54.

49. Saksena M, Gervais D. Percutaneous renal tumor ablation. Abdom Imaging 2008;34(5):582–7.

50. Cerci JJ, Pereira Neto CC, Krauzer C, et al. The impact of coaxial core biopsy guided by FDG PET/CT in oncological patients. Eur J Nucl Med Mol Imaging 2012;40(1):98–103.

51. Venkatesan AM, Kadoury S, Abi-Jaoudeh N, et al. Real-time FDG PET guidance during biopsies and radiofrequency ablation using multimodality fusion with electromagnetic navigation. Radiology 2011; 260(3):848–56.

Special Techniques in PET/Computed Tomography Imaging for Evaluation of Head and Neck Cancer

Rakesh Kumar, MD, PhD[a],*, Anirban Mukherjee, MD[a],
Bhagwant Rai Mittal, MD[b]

KEYWORDS

- ^{18}F-FDG PET/CT • Head and neck cancer • Special techniques • Open mouth • Puff cheek
- Pharmacologic intervention

KEY POINTS

- Physiologic uptake of FDG and apposed anatomic structures in head and neck can pose difficulty in interpretation of FDG PET/CT studies.
- The open-mouth and puffed-cheek techniques can depict and characterize lesions better in head and neck cancer.
- Propranolol and diazepam can help to decrease physiologic FDG uptake in the brown fat and muscle.

INTRODUCTION

Head and neck cancers (HNC) are the sixth most common cancer worldwide. An annual total of 53,640 new HNC (oral cavity, pharynx, and larynx) cases and 11,520 deaths in the United States in 2013 are reported.[1] There are many challenges in diagnosis, pretreatment staging, and posttreatment evaluation in these patients. The clinical signs and symptoms may be nonspecific and can vary depending on the tumor site in the head and neck (oral cavities, pharynx, larynx, nasal cavity, paranasal sinuses, salivary glands, thyroid, and skin). Some cancers are so occult that they escape detection by detailed physical examination, endoscopy, and conventional cross-sectional imaging.

Contrast-enhanced computed tomography (CT), MRI, and PET/CT are widely used to determine the presence and extent of the tumors before and after treatment. However, PET/CT is superior to CT and MRI in detection of carcinoma of unknown primary, cervical lymph node metastasis, distant metastasis, residual tumor, recurrent disease, and second primary tumors resulting in alteration in treatment planning.[2–5] Thus, PET with fluorodeoxyglucose F 18 (FDG)/CT plays a significant role in the management of patients with HNC in whom treatment is often expensive and associated with a significant morbidity. However, the interpretation of FDG PET/CT studies in the head and neck is challenging because of the inherently complex anatomy, physiologic variants, and unusual patterns

The authors have nothing to disclose.
[a] Diagnostic Nuclear Medicine Division, Department of Nuclear Medicine, All India Institute of Medical Sciences, New Delhi 110029, India; [b] Department of Nuclear Medicine, Post Graduate Institute of Medical Education and Research, Chandigarh 160012, India
* Corresponding author.
E-mail address: rkphulia@yahoo.com

PET Clin 11 (2016) 13–20
http://dx.doi.org/10.1016/j.cpet.2015.07.006
1556-8598/16/$ – see front matter © 2016 Elsevier Inc. All rights reserved.

of FDG uptake after radiation therapy and surgery.[6–9] Because FDG is not a tumor-specific tracer, it can accumulate in a variety of benign processes including benign tumors, inflammatory, posttraumatic, and iatrogenic conditions. In addition, there is physiologic uptake of FDG uptake in brown fat, muscles, vocal cords, and lymphatic system in the head and neck region. Lesion characterization on the CT portion of the PET/CT study is therefore of utmost importance because it increases the specificity of PET/CT reporting.[10]

However, despite its improved capabilities, PET/CT does not always accurately depict the tumor or demonstrate its margins. Apposed anatomic structures are sometimes difficult to distinguish from each other, and the exact outline of the tumor may still be undefined. In the case of a small tumor, apposition could almost hide the lesion. Moreover, during apnea and quiet respiration, the true vocal cords and the laryngeal ventricles are poorly visualized; consequently, small lesions could be misdiagnosed. In addition, examination of the oral cavity and oropharynx is often inconclusive because of dental amalgam artifacts.[11]

Physiologic uptake of FDG in areas of brown adipose tissue (BAT) and muscles of the neck also make interpretation of FDG PET/CT studies difficult.[12] In such cases, specific interventions, such as use of different dynamic maneuvers and pharmacologic interventions, may provide useful information about the lesion. These techniques facilitate providing information concerning lesion size, location, volume, and relationship with surrounding structures to the nuclear medicine physician and help to differentiate physiologic uptake of FDG from the pathologic uptake. This article reviews the use of different intervention techniques in FDG PET/CT imaging for their possible applications in head and neck imaging.

PUFFED-CHEEK TECHNIQUE
Method

This technique was recently described by Weissman and Carrau.[13] By puffing the cheeks,

the oral vestibule is filled with air, which by creating a negative contrast separates the buccal and labial mucosa from the gingival mucosa, allowing both mucosal surfaces to be assessed separately (**Figs. 1** and **2**). The buccinators muscle, the pterygomandibular raphe, and the retromolar trigone can be better delineated. Assessment of the loss of mucosal pliability caused by accompanying submucosal fibrosis is also facilitated. If during conventional FDG PET/CT acquisition focal uptake of FDG is noted in the oral cavity using the puffed-cheek maneuver, an additional PET/CT acquisition, which usually takes around 4 minutes, should be performed.

The patient is asked to close the mouth and fully puff the cheeks and breathe through the nose during the 3- to 4-minute PET/CT acquisition. It is better not to use any fluid distention or device because the puffed-cheek scanning time is relatively short and it can lead to salivation and attenuation effects.[14,15]

Indications

The puffed-cheek technique is indicated following a previous quiet respiration examination when the apposition of the buccal mucosal surface and the gingival mucosal surface hinders location and demonstration of the extent of a tumor of the oral cavity. It may also be useful when the mucosal surfaces of the tongue and the gingiva are apposed. Chang and colleagues[16] demonstrated that adopting the puffed-cheek maneuver on FDG PET/CT is practical and has several benefits for assessing oral cancer extent over conventional FDG PET/CT. In their study the accuracy in classifying localized or extended oral cancers of puffed-cheek FDG PET/CT and conventional FDG PET/CT was 95.2% and 54.5%, respectively. Puffed-cheek FDG PET/CT depicted oral cancers more accurately than conventional FDG PET/CT (P=.04) and provided preoperative assessment of the tumor thickness. Grade 3 dental artifacts on conventional FDG PET/CT images were reduced by 70% in the puffed-cheek FDG PET/CT.

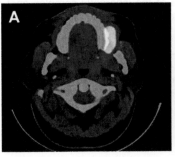 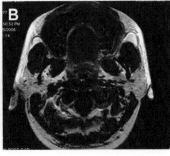

Fig. 1. A 52-year-old man presented with carcinoma of the left buccal mucosa, sent for whole-body PET/CT scan for staging. Conventional FDG PET/CT image demonstrated abnormal foci of FDG uptake in left buccal mucosa, which cannot be separated from gingival mucosa (A). Puffed-cheek view of T1-weighted MRI clearly shows a lesion in buccal mucosa extending up to retromolar trigone posteriorly (B).

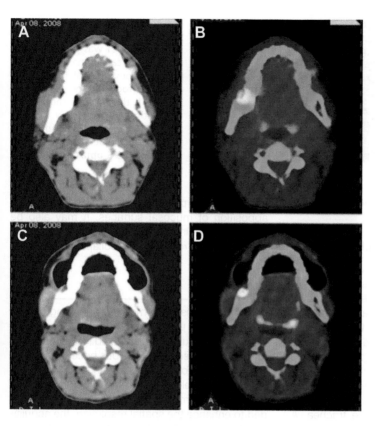

Fig. 2. A 57-year-old man presented with carcinoma of the right buccal mucosa, sent for whole-body PET/CT scan for staging. Conventional CT image showing mild thickening in the buccal mucosa (*A*), which shows increased FDG uptake in PET/CT images (*B*) but cannot be separated from gingival mucosa. Puffed-cheek view (*bottom row*) showing nodular thickening of pterygomandibular raphe and gingival mucosa clearly separates it from buccal mucosa on CT image (*C*), the same showing increased FDG uptake in PET/CT image (*D*).

Puffed-cheek FDG PET/CT could improve the assessment of oral cancer extent and delineate oral cancer better, which may provide pivotal information for planning safe margins for surgery and intensity-modulated radiation therapy (see **Figs. 1** and **2**).[17] The incremental information provided by puffed-cheek FDG PET/CT may facilitate more precise cancer targeting while reducing the normal tissue dose and adverse effects, and the overall survival rate of intensity-modulated radiation therapy seems to be similar to that of conventional radiotherapy.[18] Puffed-cheek PET/CT should be performed routinely in the clinical setting of oral cancer to improve the ability to delineate the extent and location with the additional benefit of reducing dental artifacts.

OPEN-MOUTH TECHNIQUE
Method

This technique is described by Henrot and colleagues.[11] A routine conventional whole-body FDG PET/CT was taken from supraorbital margin to mid-thigh. Then the patient is asked to open the mouth. A device (ie, a 50-mL syringe) is then placed between the teeth to ensure correct immobilization. The acquisition is performed during quiet respiration. The laser is directed to the open mouth,

and an additional 3- to 4-minute PET/CT scan is acquired from the orbitomeatal line to the clavicular fossa, with one field of view (15 cm, 3.5 minutes). CT parameters are a scan thickness of 3.75 mm, 140 kV, and 60 to 80 mA/s.[15]

Indications

The open-mouth technique is indicated when a tumor of the oral cavity and oropharynx is not clearly visible because of dental amalgam artifact. An x-ray beam crossing dental amalgam is submitted to an attenuation equivalent to that of lead filtration. Cistaro and colleagues[15] evaluate usefulness of this technique in patients with oral carcinomas. They found that for tumor localization, detection of tumor extent, and involvement of the surrounding structure open-mouth view always resulted in better scoring compared with conventional closed-mouth view (**Fig. 3**). They also found that in four patients, tumors were not detected by using the closed-mouth technique but were correctly detected using the open-mouth method because of better identification of the anatomic structures. These data suggest that compared with conventional FDG PET/CT alone, an open-mouth FDG PET/CT scan in patients with oral cavity carcinomas can improve the tumor localization,

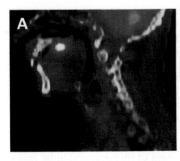
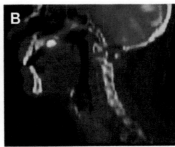

Fig. 3. A 32-year-old man presented with cervical lymph node metastases. FDG PET/CT was performed for detection of carcinoma of unknown primary. Conventional FDG PET/CT revealed foci of increased FDG uptake in the base of the tongue (A). Additional spot view of head and neck performed using open-mouth technique clearly depicts the foci of FDG uptake in the hard palate (B).

evaluation of tumor extent, and detection of tumor involvement of adjacent structures.

MODIFIED VALSALVA MANEUVER
Method

The modified Valsalva maneuver was described by Jonsson[19] in 1934 as "a method for examination of the hypopharynx and upper airway passages." Expiration is performed not against the resistance of the closed glottis but against the resistance of pursed lips or a pursed nose. The patient should be able to hold his or her breath for at least 10 seconds. Previous patient training is recommended before the examination. The scanning range is selected from the hyoid bone to the trachea. A 1-mm section thickness is recommended to enhance the spatial resolution, the acquisition is acquired within 10 seconds to avoid motion artifacts, and the pitch and table speed are selected as per Henrot and coworkers.[11] The major effects of the modified Valsalva maneuver are to open the glottis and to distend the laryngeal vestibule and piriform sinuses.[20] The true and false vocal cords are abducted and thus are generally poorly depicted. Good separation of the postcricoid and postarytenoid soft tissue from the posterior pharyngeal wall can also be achieved. Misdiagnosed small lesions of the hypopharynx and laryngeal vestibule are more easily identified. Tumor extension to the different walls of the piriform sinus is also more visible, and local staging is more accurate.

When expiration is performed against the resistance of a pursed nose, another noticeable effect is the possibility of opening the pharyngeal recess (Rosenmüller fossa) with the ability to determine whether one or two walls are invaded by a nasopharyngeal tumor. Useful information for local staging according to the TNM classification[21] is also provided by this maneuver.

Indications

The modified Valsalva maneuver is basically indicated when a previous quiet respiration examination does not correctly evaluate the location and extent of a hypopharyngeal tumor because of apposition of mucosal surfaces. It may also be useful in examination of the nasopharynx when the pharyngeal recesses are collapsed.

PHONATION
Method

This maneuver is performed by instructing the patient to say "e" uniformly for at least 10 seconds. The patient should be able to hold his or her breath for at least 10 seconds. Previous patient training is recommended before the examination. The scanning range is selected from the hyoid bone to the trachea. A 1-mm section thickness is recommended to enhance the spatial resolution, the acquisition is acquired within 10 seconds to avoid motion artifacts, and the pitch and table speed are selected as per Henrot and cowokers.[11] With phonation, the true and false vocal cords are easier to depict than with quiet respiration and the laryngeal ventricles filled with air become more visible. The true and false vocal cords are adducted and tense; consequently, abnormal thickness of a true vocal cord is more easily recognized. Visualization of the laryngeal ventricles allows more accurate determination of the location of a supraglottic tumor (above the ventricles) or a glottic tumor (below the ventricles).[11]

Indications

Phonation is indicated when the true and false vocal cords are not clearly depicted and when the exact location of a laryngeal tumor remains undefined following a quiet respiration examination. The true vocal cords could be apposed and indistinguishable from one another when the acquisition is performed during apnea. However, they may be abducted and thus not visible when the acquisition is performed during quiet respiration.[11]

Modified Valsalva and phonation maneuvers are mainly used during CT acquisition. Performing hybrid PET/CT with these two maneuvers is difficult because PET acquisition even for one field of view requires a minimum time duration of 2 to

3 minutes. It is extremely difficult to perform modified Valsalva or phonation technique for this period. Thus, there are motion artifact and difficulty in coregistration of CT and PET images. However, when there is abnormal focus of uptake noted in the hypopharynx or larynx during conventional PET/CT acquisition an additional CT acquisition using this technique should be performed and reviewed along with conventional whole-body PET/CT.

PHARMACOLOGIC INTERVENTION
β-Blockers

Propranolol, a nonselective β-adrenergic receptor-blocking agent, can be used to reduce FDG uptake in the BAT, which is one of the most common cause of false-positive study during FDG acquisition. BAT is generally present in deep cervical regions, including the supraclavicular areas, the interscapular and paravertebral regions, and areas near large vessels. Areas of involvement are often spatially closely related to important lymph node groups in the neck, axilla, and upper mediastinum, making critical differentiation difficult. The uptake of FDG in BAT limits the ability of a PET scan to detect the sites of viable disease. BAT is a highly specialized thermogenic tissue that plays an important role in the regulation of body temperature in newborn and hibernating mammals.[22] It also plays an important role in cold-induced and diet-induced thermogenesis.[23] Morphologically, BAT differs from regular or white adipose tissue by its rich vascularization and its high density of mitochondria. These features are responsible for its brownish color.[24]

The function of BAT is to generate heat; this function is triggered by the sympathetic nervous system. BAT expresses $β_1$-, $β_2$-, and $β_3$-adrenergic receptors, among which the $β_3$-adrenergic receptor is predominant. Noradrenaline released from sympathetic nerve terminals binds to $β_3$-receptors on the surfaces of BAT cells and causes, in a cyclic adenosine monophosphate–mediated process, activation of the enzyme hormone-sensitive lipase. Hormone-sensitive lipase degrades cytoplasmic triglycerides, and the free fatty acids generated from this process enter β-oxidation in the mitochondria and initiate heat production.[22] In addition, noradrenaline activates glucose transport by glucose transporter 1 and potentially also by glucose transporter 4 in an insulin-independent manner.[25,26] This explains the biologic mechanism underlying the accumulation of FDG in activated BAT.[27–30]

Propranolol being a nonselective β-blocker blocks $β_3$-receptors and causes decrease in the FDG uptake (**Fig. 4**). In a study performed by Agarwal and colleagues,[12] they demonstrated that 40 mg of propranolol administered orally 60 minutes before FDG PET/CT acquisition can successfully eliminate FDG activity from the BAT.

Benzodiazepine

Use of benzodiazepines can also decrease FDG uptake in BAT. Barrington and Maisey[31] found significantly decreased BAT uptake by using 5 to 10 mg of diazepam orally 30 to 60 minutes before intravenous administration of FDG. It was suggested that in humans the central antianxiety effect of diazepam may relieve the sympathetic nervous system activity and thus reduce FDG uptake in BAT. However, use of benzodiazepines is associated with significant side effects. Furthermore, some other authors found little value in using diazepam as a premedication for suppression of brown fat.[32,33] Thus, it is not recommended for routine use.

Benzodiazepines can also be used during head and neck imaging to decrease muscle uptake. Physiologic FDG uptake is often seen in the muscles of the head and neck, which can constitute a diagnostic dilemma in the interpretation of PET scans.[6–9,34–36] Prominent physiologic uptake can be seen in the tongue and in the pterygoid muscles on vocalization and chewing after FDG injection. Prominent FDG uptake is also often seen in the extraocular muscles because of eye motion. In the neck, physiologic FDG uptake can be seen in the visceral and nonvisceral compartment musculature. In the visceral compartment, pronounced uptake in the cricopharyngeus and posterior cricoarytenoid muscles on phonation can interfere with the interpretation of PET scans in patients with hypopharyngeal, esophageal, and thyroid cancers, in whom this physiologic uptake may mimic pathology.[6,34,36,37] Uptake in the anterior portion of the genioglossus muscles can mimic or obscure small floor of the mouth cancers. Contraction-induced increased FDG uptake in the cervical muscles, strap muscles, and paraspinal muscles in anxious patients (in particular sternocleidomastoid, scalenus anterior, longus colli, longus capitis, and inferior obliquus capiti muscles) can mimic lymph node metastasis or, alternatively, may lead to false-negative findings obscuring disease truly present in underlying lymph nodes.[6–9,34–36,38,39] Uptake in the anterior scalenus muscle mimicking supraclavicular lymph node metastasis in a case of lung cancer has been described.[39] Administration of benzodiazepines before FDG PET/CT study decreases the

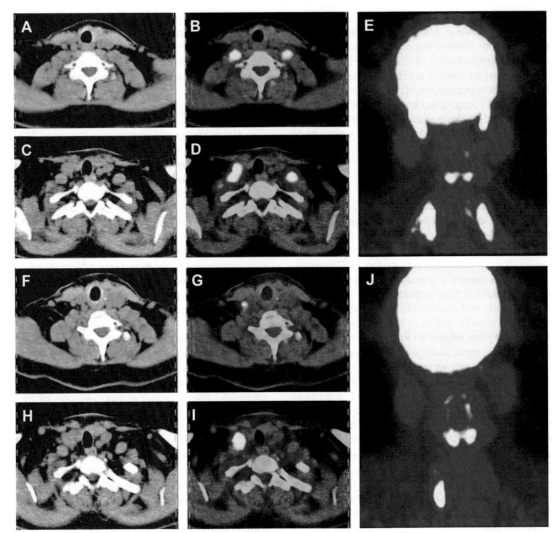

Fig. 4. A 49-year-old man with known thyroid cancer with negative I-131 whole-body scan and elevated thyroglobulin was referred for FDG PET/CT for detection of recurrent thyroid cancer. FDG PET/CT images (*A–E*) show increased FDG uptake mainly in the brown fat, bilateral pterygoid muscles masking cervical lymph nodes. The study was repeated using 40 mg of propranolol 60 minutes before intravenous FDG injection. FDG PET/CT images after propranolol (*F–J*) clearly demonstrate suppression of FDG uptake in the brown fat and neck muscle. Right-sided level IV and supraclavicular lymph nodes are clearly outlined, which were masked earlier.

muscle uptake and helps the physician in proper interpretation of the study.[40]

OPTIMIZATION OF PATIENT PREPARATION

Optimization of scan protocol can help to decrease physiologic uptake of FDG in the head and neck region. Tongue movement or sucking actions may increase FDG uptake in pharyngeal muscles.[41] Because the genioglossus muscle prevents the tongue from falling back and obstructing the airway when the body is supine, uptake in the tongue base muscles and anterior part of the floor of the mouth is higher in patients resting supine for a long time (eg, after a night's rest).[42] Oral activity, such as speaking during the waiting time between the injection and whole-body scan, increases FDG activity in the laryngeal muscles.[43] Different uptake at the level of the orbicular muscles of the mouth, lateral pterygoid, and masseter muscles can be observed if the patient chews gum during the long wait time.[44] To avoid this fallacious uptake the PET/CT examinations can be scheduled around mid-morning to avoid the possibility of supine position–related FDG uptake in the muscles at the base of the tongue and anterior part of the mouth floor. Patients should fast for at least 6 hours before examination and be instructed to remain silent and abstain from liquid intake 30 minutes before the injection and during the waiting time between FDG injection and whole-body scanning to avoid FDG uptake by the tongue and vocal muscles. During this period, patients should not be allowed to lie down. Before the scan, all metal objects (eg, necklaces, earrings, and prosthesis) are removed to avoid metal attenuation artifacts. Cistaro and colleagues[15] evaluated the use of this optimization of patient preparation in patients with HNC. They found significant suppression of the muscle uptake using this patient preparation protocol. If this method is followed meticulously significant reduction in FDG uptake in the muscles of base of tongue and floor of the mouth can be achieved.

SUMMARY

FDG PET/CT imaging has dramatically changed HCN imaging and management. FDG, however, is not tumor-specific and various image interpretation pitfalls may occur because of false-positive and -negative causes of FDG uptake. In some cases, routine imaging examination of head and neck malignancies does not yield all of the necessary data, even with the most advanced imaging technique. Additional scans obtained with dynamic maneuvers can depict some lesions that were previously nonidentified because of apposition of anatomic structures or the presence of dental amalgam artifacts. The open-mouth technique, puffed-cheek technique, modified Valsalva maneuver, and phonation should be performed in these situations. Use of certain premedication, such as propranolol and diazepam, can help to decrease physiologic FDG uptake in the brown fat and muscle. Optimal patient preparation technique can also help to decrease FDG uptake in the base of the tongue and floor of the mouth. However, use of these additional spot views is associated with increased radiation exposure and use of premedication can lead to certain side effects. These should be carefully weighed against the expected improvement of the diagnostic value; therefore, these interventions should be performed only after conventional whole-body FDG PET/CT examination with inconclusive results.

REFERENCES

1. Siegel R, Naishadham D, Jemal A. Cancer statistics, 2013. CA Cancer J Clin 2013;63:11–30.
2. Ha PK, Hdeib A, Goldenberg D, et al. The role of positron emission tomography and computed tomography fusion in the management of early-stage and advanced-stage primary head and neck squamous cell carcinoma. Arch Otolaryngol Head Neck Surg 2006;132:12–6.
3. Miller FR, Hussey D, Beeram M, et al. Positron emission tomography in the management of unknown primary head and neck carcinoma. Arch Otolaryngol Head Neck Surg 2005;131:626–9.
4. Gupta T, Master Z, Kannan S, et al. Diagnostic performance of post-treatment FDG PET or FDG PET/CT imaging in head and neck cancer: a systematic review and meta-analysis. Eur J Nucl Med Mol Imaging 2011;38:2083–95.
5. Scott AM, Gunawardana DH, Bartholomeusz D, et al. PET changes management and improves prognostic stratification in patients with head and neck cancer: results of a multicenter prospective study. J Nucl Med 2008;49:1593–600.
6. Kostakoglu L, Hardoff R, Mirtcheva R, et al. PET-CT fusion imaging in differentiating physiologic from pathologic FDG uptake. Radiographics 2004;24:1411–31.
7. El-Haddad G, Alavi A, Mavi A, et al. Normal variants in [18 F]-fluorodeoxyglucose PET imaging. Radiol Clin North Am 2004;42:1063–81.
8. Bhargava P, Rahman S, Wendt J. Atlas of confounding factors in head and neck PET/CT imaging. Clin Nucl Med 2011;36:e20–9.
9. Castaigne C, Muylle K, Flamen P. Positron emission tomography in head and neck cancer. In: Hermans R, editor. Head and neck cancer imaging. Berlin: Springer; 2006. p. 329–43.
10. Metser U, Miller E, Lerman H, et al. Benign nonphysiologic lesions with increased 18 F-FDG uptake on PET/CT: characterization and incidence. AJR Am J Roentgenol 2007;189:1203–10.
11. Henrot P, Blum A, Toussaint B, et al. Dynamic maneuvers in local staging of head and neck malignancies with current imaging techniques: principles and clinical applications. Radiographics 2003;23(5): 1201–13.
12. Agarwal A, Nair N, Baghel NS. A novel approach for reduction of brown fat uptake on FDG PET. Br J Radiol 2009;82(980):626–31.
13. Weissman JL, Carrau RL. "Puffed-cheek" CT improves evaluation of the oral cavity. AJNR Am J Neuroradiol 2001;22:741–4.
14. Fatterpekar GM, Delman BN, Shroff MM, et al. Distension technique to improve computed tomographic evaluation of oral cavity lesions. Arch Otolaryngol Head Neck Surg 2003;129:229–32.
15. Cistaro A, Palandri S, Balsamo V, et al. Assessment of a new 18F-FDG PET/CT protocol in the staging of oral cavity carcinomas. J Nucl Med Technol 2011; 39:7–13.
16. Chang CY, Yang BH, Lin KH, et al. Feasibility and incremental benefit of puffed-cheek 18F -FDG PET/CT on oral cancer patients. Clin Nucl Med 2013;38(10): e374–8.

17. Kao CH, Hsieh TC, Yu CY, et al. 18F-FDG PET/CT-based gross tumor volume definition for radiotherapy in head and neck cancer: a correlation study between suitable uptake value threshold and tumor parameters. Radiat Oncol 2010;5:76.

18. Gomez DR, Zhung JE, Gomez J, et al. Intensity-modulated radiotherapy in postoperative treatment of oral cavity cancers. Int J Radiat Oncol Biol Phys 2009;73:1096–103.

19. Jonsson G. A method for examination of the hypopharynx and upper way passages. Acta Radiol 1934;15:125.

20. Hillel AD, Schwartz AN. Trumpet maneuver for visual and CT examination of the pyriform sinus and retrocricoid area. Head Neck 1989;11:231–6.

21. Sobin LH, Wittekind C, editors. UICC/TNM classification of malignant tumors. 5th edition. New York: Wiley; 1997.

22. Cannon B, Nedergaard J. Brown adipose tissue: function and physiological significance. Physiol Rev 2004;84:277–359.

23. Del Mar Gonzalez-Barroso M, Ricquier D, Cassard-Doulcier AM. The human uncoupling protein-1 gene (UCP1): present status and perspectives in obesity research. Obes Rev 2000;1:61–72.

24. Weber WA. Brown adipose tissue and nuclear medicine imaging. J Nucl Med 2004;45:1101–3.

25. Shimizu Y, Satoh S, Yano H, et al. Effects of noradrenaline on the cell-surface glucose transporters in cultured brown adipocytes: novel mechanism for selective activation of GLUT1 glucose transporters. Biochem J 1998;330:397–403.

26. Chernogubova E, Cannon B, Bengtsson T. Norepinephrine increases glucose transport in brown adipocytes via beta3-adrenoceptors through a cAMP, PKA, and PI3-kinase dependent pathway stimulating conventional and novel PKCs. Endocrinology 2004;145:269–80.

27. Hany TF, Gharehpapagh E, Kamel EM, et al. Brown adipose tissue: a factor to consider in symmetrical tracer uptake in the neck and upper chest region. Eur J Nucl Med Mol Imaging 2002;29:1393–8.

28. Cohade C, Osman M, Pannu HK, et al. Uptake in supraclavicular area fat ("USA-Fat"): description on 18FFDG PET/CT. J Nucl Med 2003;44:170–6.

29. Cohade C, Mourtzikos KA, Wahl RL. "USA-fat": prevalence is related to ambient outdoor temperature-evaluation with 18F-FDG PET/CT. J Nucl Med 2003;44:1267–70.

30. Yeung HW, Grewal RK, Gonen M, et al. Patterns of (18)F-FDG uptake in adipose tissue and muscle: a potential source of false-positives for PET. J Nucl Med 2003;44:1789–96.

31. Barrington SF, Maisey MN. Skeletal muscle uptake of fluorine-18-FDG: effect of oral diazepam. J Nucl Med 1996;37:1127–9.

32. Gelfand MJ, O'hara SM, Curtwright LA, et al. Premedication to block [(18)] FDG uptake in brown adipose tissue of pediatric and adolescent patients. Pediatr Radiol 2005;35:984–90.

33. Christensen CR, Clark PB, Morton KA. Reversal of hypermetabolic brown adipose tissue in F-18 FDG PET imaging. Clin Nucl Med 2006;31:193–6.

34. Blodgett TM, Fukui MB, Snyderman CH, et al. Combined PET-CT in the head and neck. Part 1: physiologic, altered physiologic, and artifactual FDG uptake. Radiographics 2005;25:897–912.

35. Fukui MB, Blodgett TM, Snyderman CH, et al. Combined PET-CT in the head and neck. Part 2: diagnostic pitfalls of oncologic imaging. Radiographics 2005;25:913–30.

36. Schöder H. Head and neck cancer. In: Strauss HW, Mariani G, Volterrani D, et al, editors. Nuclear oncology: pathophysiology and clinical applications. New York: Springer; 2013. p. 269–95.

37. Zhu Z, Chou C, Yen TC, et al. Elevated F-18 FDG uptake in laryngeal muscles mimicking thyroid cancer metastases. Clin Nucl Med 2001;26:689–91.

38. Jacene HA, Goudarzi B, Wahl RL. Scalene muscle uptake: a potential pitfall in head and neck PET/CT. Eur J Nucl Med Mol Imaging 2008;35:89–94.

39. Su HC, Huang CK, Bai YL, et al. Physiologically variant FDG uptake in scalene muscle mimicking neck lymph node metastasis in a patient with lung cancer. Ann Nucl Med Sci 2009;22:239–43.

40. Purohit BS, Ailianou A, Dulguerov N, et al. FDG-PET/CT pitfalls in oncological head and neck imaging. Insights Imaging 2014;5(5):585–602.

41. Kubota K. From tumor biology to clinical PET: a review of positron emission tomography (PET) in oncology. Ann Nucl Med 2001;15:471–86.

42. Abouzied MM, Crawford ES, Nabi AN. 18F-FDG imaging: pitfalls and artifacts. J Nucl Med Technol 2005;33:145–55.

43. Kostakoglu L, Wong JCH, Barrington SF, et al. Speech-related visualization of laryngeal muscles with florine-18-FDG. J Nucl Med 1996;37:1771–3.

44. Rikimaru H, Kikuchi M, Itoh M, et al. Mapping energy metabolism in jaw and tongue muscles during chewing. J Dent Res 2001;80:1849–53.

Recent Advances in Imaging of Small and Large Bowel

Chandan J. Das, MD[a],*, Smita Manchanda, MD[a], Ananya Panda, MD[a],
Anshul Sharma, MD[b], Arun K. Gupta, MD[a]

KEYWORDS

- Multidetector CT • MR imaging • PET-CT • Enterography • Colography

KEY POINTS

- With the advances in cross-sectional imaging, bowel imaging has reached a new zenith.
- Multidetector computed tomography (CT) is a frequently used modality because of its ease of performance in a few seconds as well as its easy availability these days.
- MR imaging is particularly useful in pediatric patients and in conditions like inflammatory bowel disease (IBD) whereby frequent imaging is necessary to avoid CT- or fluoroscopy-associated radiation.
- Present-generation PET-CT or PET-MR imaging hybrid scanners combine the functional information of PET with state-of-the-art CT or MR imaging to provide information about disease activity with precise anatomic localization.

INTRODUCTION

The diagnosis of bowel pathologic conditions is challenging in view of the nonspecific clinical presentation. Currently, there are various imaging modalities available to reach an accurate diagnosis. These modalities include conventional techniques (radiographs, small bowel follow-through, conventional enteroclysis), ultrasonography (US), and cross-sectional examinations (computed tomography [CT] and MR imaging) as well as functional imaging modalities, such as PET-CT or PET-MR imaging. Each modality has its own advantages and disadvantages and can be used in isolation or combination. This review discusses the role of CT, MR imaging, and PET-CT in the evaluation of small and large bowel diseases.

EVALUATION OF THE BOWEL

Conventional radiographs (erect and supine) are now mainly used for an initial diagnosis of obstruction and perforation of the bowel. In case of a suspected subacute intestinal obstruction, the radiographs need to be performed during the acute episode. Chest radiograph is an inexpensive tool to detect pneumoperitoneum as gas under the diaphragm.

Small bowel follow-through and conventional enteroclysis can well depict intraluminal pathology; however, they have radiation exposure and are unable to evaluate bowel wall and extraluminal disease.[1]

Bowel wall thickening can be well visualized with US without any risk of radiation exposure.

Conflict of interests: none.
[a] Department of Radiology, All India Institute of Medical Sciences, New Delhi 110029, India; [b] Department of Nuclear Medicine, All India Institute of Medical Sciences, Ansari Nagar, New Delhi 110029, India
* Corresponding author.
E-mail address: dascj@yahoo.com

pet.theclinics.com

However, it is difficult to evaluate all the loops or make an etiologic diagnosis. Moreover, it is operator dependent and difficult to perform in acute state as well as in obese patient.

CROSS-SECTIONAL IMAGING
Computed Tomography

CT-based methods include abdominal CT (unenhanced and enhanced), CT enteroclysis (CTEc), CT enterography (CTE), and CT colonography (CTC).

Routine Computed Tomography Abdomen

Unenhanced and contrast-enhanced CT abdomen is a routine procedure and can be performed in emergency and post-trauma settings. Images are acquired from the diaphragm to the symphysis pubis in the portal venous phase after the administration of intravenous nonionic iodinated contrast. Positive oral contrast material is given in the form of 1% to 2% barium sulfate or 2% to 3% iodine-based solution. These positive agents help in the differentiation of bowel loops and for determining pathology as intraluminal or extraluminal. However, these interfere in the evaluation of intestinal wall characteristics and angiography images.[2] Positive contrast materials should not be used in patients with suspicious vascular disease and clinical presentation of gastrointestinal (GI) bleeding.

Negative oral contrast agents like lactulose, water, oil emulsion, methylcellulose, polyethylene glycol (PEG), mannitol, and ultra–low-dose barium with sorbitol (volumen) are preferred in the assessment of intestinal wall enhancement. However, it is difficult to evaluate hypodense lesions like abscess and cyst.[3]

CTEc is performed after nasojejunal intubation under fluoroscopy. As this process is invasive for patients and requires an extra tube, CTE is the preferred technique these days. For this 300 mL 20% w/v mannitol is mixed with 1.5 L water. A total of 500 mL of mixture is given orally to patients in the first 15 minutes followed by 500 mL in the next 15 minutes, then 500 mL in the next 15 minutes. The scan is performed at 50 minutes with the remaining solution given on the table along with intravenous contrast injection to patient (**Box 1**).

Computed Tomographic Colonography

CTC is easy to perform and is less invasive than colonoscopy. The details of the technique are summarized in **Box 2**.

> **Box 1**
> **CT enteroclysis**
>
> Fasting: at least 8 hours of fasting before the examination
>
> Intestine cleansing: 1 day before all of the enteroclysis and enterographic examinations with 50 to 100 mL of laxative diet solution (polyethylene glycol)
>
> Acquisition: from the diaphragm to the symphysis pubis
>
> Intravenous contrast agent: 100 mL nonionic
>
> Portal venous phase: images obtained 50 seconds after the administration of contrast material (flow rate, 4 mL/s; total 150 mL)
>
> Oral contrast: 300 mL 20% wt/vol mannitol mixed with 1.5 L water

PET with Fludeoxyglucose F 18/Computed Tomography

PET with fludeoxyglucose F 18 ([18]FDG-PET)/CT has rapidly obtained a foothold in the evaluation of bowel disorders, chiefly in neoplasms and inflammatory bowel diseases (IBDs). [18]FDG-PET imaging relies on the increased uptake and metabolism of [18]FDG in inflammation, infection, or neoplasm.[4,5] Combining [18]FDG-PET with CT, both morphologic and functional information regarding disease site and activity can be obtained. This imaging technique has been enhanced further by combining CTE/CTEc and CTC with [18]FDG-PET imaging for the evaluation of the small and large bowel, respectively.[6,7]

Technique of PET with Fludeoxyglucose F 18/Computed Tomography Enterography

For [18]FDG-PET/CTE, patients are asked to come with 6 to 8 hours of fasting and intestinal preparation similar to that for CTE. The blood glucose is checked for hyperglycemia, and [18]FDG is administered either at a fixed dose of 10 mCi or as a weight-based dose (0.15 mCi/kg) in the pediatric population. For PET-CTE, patients are asked to drink 1.5 L of mannitol solution over 45 minutes to 50 minutes, whereas for PET-CTEc, a nasojejunal tube is inserted up to the proximal jejunum and 1.5 L of normal saline is given through it until patients complain of abdominal distension/discomfort. The [18]FDG-PET/CTE scanning begins 45 minutes to 60 minutes after injection of [18]FDG. Initially a low-dose CT is obtained from the domes of the diaphragm to the pubic symphysis followed by [18]FDG-PET imaging, and the data obtained from CTE are used for attenuation correction for [18]FDG-PET. The authors do not administer

---

Box 2
CTC

Bowel preparation

1. Low-fiber diet for 1 to 3 days

2. Bowel purgation: polyethylene glycol

3. Fecal tagging: oral administration of either water-soluble iodinated contrast medium or a diluted barium sulfate suspension, which is done to tag residual bowel content and differentiate from true colonic lesions

Colonic distension

Colon is inflated with air or carbon dioxide by using a thin and flexible rectal catheter.

Image acquisition

Noncontrast images: prone position

Contrast-enhanced CT: supine position

Intravenous administration of 100 mL of nonionic contrast

Portal venous phase acquisition

Optimal colonic distension: if the entire colonic wall is pencil-thin with thin haustral folds

Analysis of axial and reformatted images

Use of computer-aided detection software

Data from Laghi A. Computed tomography colonography in 2014: an update on technique and indications. World J Gastroenterol 2014;20(45):16858–67; and Narayanan S, Kalra N, Bhatia A, et al. Staging of colorectal cancer using contrast-enhanced multidetector computed tomographic colonography. Singapore Med J 2014;55(12):660–6.

---

intravenous iodinated contrast routinely while performing this procedure.

Technique of PET with Fludeoxyglucose F 18/Computed Tomography Colonography

Two techniques of colonic distension have been described when CTC is combined with [18]FDG-PET imaging.[7,8] In the authors' institute, they obtain adequate colonic distension by giving the patients 2.5 to 4.0 L of water mixed with 2 packets of polyethylene glycol (each packet containing 137.5 mg polyethylene glycol) perorally. Patients are asked to drink this slowly over a period of 1 hour, and scanning is done 45 minutes to 60 minutes after intravenous injection of [18]FDG. This technique provides adequate colonic distension without the invasiveness of rectal injection. Other authors have obtained colonic distension by per-rectal injection of 2 to 3 L of tap water.[8] Colonic distension takes less time with this technique albeit with the discomfort of an enema preparation.

PET with Fludeoxyglucose F 18/Computed Tomography Radiation Issues

Although the functional information provided by [18]FDG-PET/CT is a useful addition to anatomic cross-sectional imaging techniques in evaluation of bowel, radiation dose is an important issue in PET/CT imaging. As most patients with IBD are

young patients who require long-term follow-up, optimizing the use of this imaging technique is important. With older scanners, the radiation dose with whole-body PET/CT was approximately 25 mSv, 18 mSv for the CT, and 7 mSv for PET scanning. However, this dose can be decreased with the following measures. Firstly, in a known case of IBD, the whole-body PET/CT can be replaced by limited CT covering only the abdomen and pelvis.[9] Secondly, the tube current and kilovoltage parameters can be decreased during CT scanning, especially in pediatric cases.[10] Thirdly, newer scanners have automatic dose modulation software, which can automatically decrease the tube current according to thickness of different body areas.[11] Fourthly, iterative-based reconstruction algorithms can obtain diagnostic quality images with equivalent noise at lesser tube currents and can provide up to 40% dose reduction.[12] Lastly, rather than using a fixed dose of [18]FDG PET radiopharmaceutical, a weight-based dose can decrease the radiation exposure to patients, especially for thinner and younger patients. PET-MR imaging also holds promise, as MR imaging is free of radiation along with new low-dose PET.

MR Imaging

MR imaging–related procedures include routine MR imaging abdomen, magnetic resonance (MR) enteroclysis, and MR enterography. MR imaging is now increasingly being used for the evaluation of bowel pathology in view of the lack of ionizing radiation and superior contrast resolution. The reduction in radiation exposure is significant for patients with chronic IBD (especially the pediatric age group) who need repeated evaluation. The other advantages over CT include the ability to use it in pregnancy and in patients with an allergy to iodine-based contrast agents.[13]

The potential disadvantages include longer acquisition times, higher cost, and motion artifacts. Motion artifacts can be eliminated partially with the use of fast sequences and antispasmodic agents, such as hyoscine, which decreases bowel movement.[14]

Although MR enteroclysis provides better mucosal detail,[15,16] it involves nasojejunal intubation, which is an invasive procedure and involves ionizing radiation during fluoroscopy-guided tube insertion.[17] MR enterography (MRE) is currently the preferred technique as it is faster and more tolerable (**Box 3**).

MR imaging protocol includes axial and coronal T2 weighted image for an overview of the wall thickness of the intestinal segments and existing edema. Coronal balanced steady state free precession sequence is acquired in the axial and coronal plane for extraintestinal changes, such as mesenteric lymph nodes or vascular hyperemia. Noncontrast T1-weighted sequences are acquired

for large bowel evaluation as it can allow possible contrast-enhanced polyps to be differentiated from stool residue (hyperintense in noncontrast sequences). Dynamic contrast-enhanced acquisition is performed, and fat-saturated T1 turbo spin echo sequences are obtained in the axial and coronal planes during the late phase following administration of contrast medium[20] (**Fig. 1**).

Diffusion-Weighted Imaging

Diffusion-weighted imaging (DWI) can help to identify pathologic segments (in patients with chronic IBDs) and grade the severity of disease by apparent diffusion coefficient (ADC) values[21,22] (**Fig. 2**). It can also detect any additional inflammatory or tumorous lesions. This sequence is advantageous in patients with renal failure, as it does not involve contrast medium administration. Because of the faster acquisition, it can easily be added to routine evaluation protocol.[23]

Interpretation of Bowel Pathology on Cross-sectional Imaging

The normal bowel

Wall thickness may vary according to the degree of distension of bowel. The small bowel wall should not be more than 3 mm thick even in maximal luminal distention, whereas in the large bowel, thickness can vary from 1 to 2 mm in the distended state to 5 mm in the nondistended

---

Box 3
MR enterography

Fasting: at least 8 hours

Intestinal clearing: polyethylene glycol

Antispasmodic: 1 mL (10 mg) hyoscine butylbromide intravenously after initial localized sequence and another 1 mL hyoscine butylbromide before injecting gadolinium

Contrast agents:

1. Positive (bright lumen): hyperintense on T1-weighted and T2-weighted images, gadolinium-chelates, ferrous/manganese ions, milk, blueberry juice, green tea, and ice cream[3]; used for the evaluation of the passage of contrast material through the bowel loops

2. Negative (dark lumen): hypointense on T1-weighted and T2-weighted images; ferumoxsil oral suspension, oral supermagnetic particles, and perfluorooctyl-bromide[18]

3. Biphasic contrast agents (water-based): hyperintense on T2-weighted and hypointense on T1-weighted sequences; water, diatrizoate meglumine, diatrizoate sodium salt, mannitol, locust bean gum, low-dose barium, manganese compounds, and PEG[16]; usually preferred as the luminal hypointensity on T1-weighted images helps to differentiate it from wall enhancement/mass and better vascular assessment[3]

Position:

1. Prone position preferred to facilitate separation of small bowel loops and minimize respiratory excursion, has added advantage of shorter acquisition time as volume of peritoneal cavity to be imaged decreases, hence, lesser number of coronal sections needed[19]

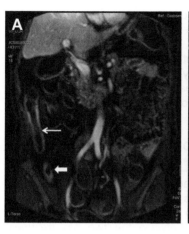
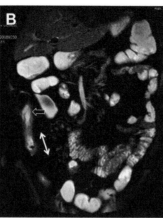

Fig. 1. MR imaging post–gadolinium-enhanced coronal image (A) shows abnormal long segment enhancement of ascending colon (*white arrow*) and distal ileum (*block arrow*). Steady-state precession coronal image (B) shows long segment wall thickening (*black block arrow*) and mesenteric hyperemia (*double arrow*) or comb's sign suggestive of active inflammation.

state.[24] The valvulae conniventes should be less than 3 mm thick, and the caliber of small intestine should be less than 3 cm.[2] The bowel wall normally enhances after the administration of intravenous contrast material.

The enterographic images should be evaluated for the intestinal caliber and distribution and thickness of the valvulae conniventes. The thickness of the bowel wall, pattern of thickening, and enhancement also help to narrow the differential diagnosis. An assessment of the mesentery, lymph nodes, and other viscera should also be made on CTE or MRE.[2] The abnormal small bowel can be approached by looking into pattern of

enhancement, length of involvement, degree of thickening, pattern of thickening (symmetric or asymmetric), location of the lesion along the course of the small bowel (proximal or distal), location of the lesion in the wall of the small bowel (mucosal, submucosal, or serosal), and associated abnormalities in the mesentery and vessels.[25]

PATHOLOGIC ABNORMALITIES
Tuberculosis

Tuberculosis (TB) commonly involves the bowel, with the ileocecal junction being the most frequently affected. TB of the bowel can be of

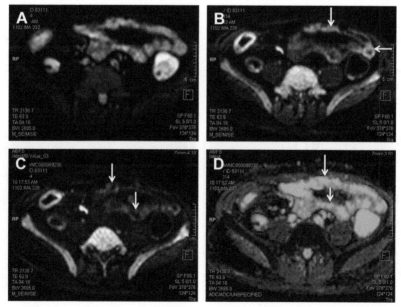

Fig. 2. Diffusion-weighted axial images at b values 0 (A), 400 (B), and 80 (C) show progressive increase in signal intensity of abnormal and thickened bowel wall (*white arrows*), which are dark on the corresponding ADC map (*white arrows*, D) suggestive of restricted diffusion.

4 types: ulcerative, hypertrophic, ulcerohypertrophic, and fibrous stricturing. In the ulcerative type, there are shallow ulcers better seen on the barium studies. Exophytic masses around the ulcerated lumen are seen in the hypertrophic and ulcerohypertrophic forms (**Fig. 3**). Fibrous stricturing causes shortening, retraction, and occasional annular growths, which mimic malignancy.[26]

Cross-sectional imaging reveals bowel wall thickening, especially in the ileocecal region involving the ileocecal valve and medial wall of caecum (**Fig. 4**). It may be mild and symmetric or severe and asymmetric with heterogeneous areas (**Fig. 5**). Exophytic masses may be seen surrounding a narrowed, ulcerated lumen. There are associated necrotic enlarged mesenteric and retroperitoneal lymph nodes. Omental nodularity, peritoneal thickening, and free fluid may be seen in the abdomen.[27]

Crohn disease (CD) is an important differential of TB enteritis (**Box 4**). In CD there is less marked and circumferential wall thickening with preserved mural stratification. In addition, lymph nodes are of soft tissue density, and the omentum and peritoneum are normal. The fibrofatty proliferation and comb sign characteristic of CD are not seen in TB. Fistula and sinus tract formation are also more frequently observed in CD.[26]

Malabsorption Syndromes

These syndromes include conditions like celiac disease, tropical sprue, Whipple disease, and intestinal lymphangiectasia.[2] Celiac disease is characterized by chronic inflammation due to sensitivity to gluten with resultant atrophy of the intestinal villi. On cross-sectional imaging, there is small bowel dilatation, mesenteric hyperemia, and reversed jejunoileal fold pattern. This reversal is best seen on coronal reformatted images of CTE or coronal sequences in MR enterography, as a

decrease in jejunal folds and increasing fold pattern of the ileum.[28] In addition, mesenteric engorgement, mesenteric and retroperitoneal lymphadenopathy, transient intussusception, and splenic atrophy can be demonstrated in patients with celiac disease.[29] CT-MR imaging can also depict complications like development of lymphoma/malignancy.

INFLAMMATORY BOWEL DISEASES
Crohn Disease

CD is an idiopathic chronic inflammatory disease, which involves all layers of the bowel wall. It can present in active or chronic phase or both. Differentiation between the two has treatment implications as active inflammation is managed medically, whereas chronic fibrostenoses needs surgical intervention.[28]

Cross-sectional imaging can demonstrate the features of active and chronic disease and any associated complications. There is long segment wall thickening associated with increased mucosal enhancement and bowel wall edema in active disease (see **Fig. 1**; **Fig. 6**). Increased mesenteric vascularity seen as the comb sign, perienteric inflammation (**Fig. 7**), increased attenuation of the terminal ileum, and enlarged mesenteric lymph nodes are the associated findings.[30] Ulcerations can be picked up on T2-weighted MR imaging as longitudinal or transverse linear hyperintensities within the thickened bowel wall.

Strictures may be seen in active phase as luminal narrowing associated with wall thickening, mucosal hyperenhancement, and inflammatory spasm.

In the chronic stage, there is mural fibrosis leading to stricture formation and aperistalsis of the bowel loop on MR fluoroscopy. The thickened wall in this chronic phase is hypointense on T2-weighted images with reduced enhancement

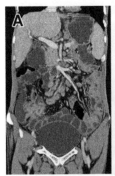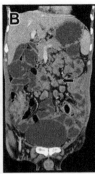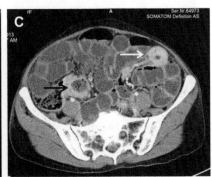

Fig. 3. CTE coronal (*A, B*) and axial (*C*) images in patient with TB show thickening involving terminal ileum and ileocecal junction (*black arrow, C*). There is also separate focus of wall thickening and enhancement in proximal ileum (*white arrow, C*) and mesenteric nodes (*block arrow, B*).

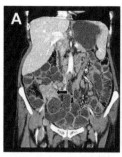
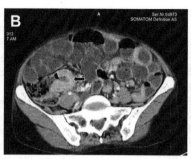
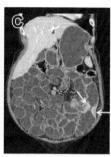

Fig. 4. CTE coronal (*A, C*) and axial images of a known case (the same patient in **Fig. 3**) of TB show multifocal wall thickening involving both distal ileum (*block arrows; A, B*) and jejunum (*white arrows, C*). There is also focal narrowing in jejunum (*C*). These findings are suggestive of the ulcerohypertrophic form of TB and closely mimics Crohn disease.

and loss of mural stratification. Submucosal fat deposition, fibrofatty proliferation, and sacculations of the antimesenteric wall are other features of chronic disease.

In the fistulizing-penetrating subtype, there are deep ulcers with transmural extension. This condition leads to the formation of abscesses and sinus or fistula formation with adjacent bowel loops or other organs. The presence of bowel angulation with linear tracts between the bowel loops is suggestive of fistula formation. Fistulas are seen as T2 hyperintense tracts, which are hyperenhancing after contrast administration. Abscesses are seen commonly in the retroperitoneum and mesentery as extraluminal fluid collections and can be drained under ultrasound or CT guidance.[28]

Cross-sectional imaging also helps to evaluate the extraintestinal manifestations like hepatobiliary (sclerosing cholangitis, cholelithiasis, liver abscess, portal vein thrombosis), renal (hydronephrosis, nephrolithiasis), and peritoneal pseudocysts.[31]

Ulcerative Colitis

Ulcerative colitis (UC) is an IBD involving the colonic mucosa. In 95% of the cases, there is rectal involvement with variable proximal involvement.[32] It may be associated with backwash ileitis in which the ileocecal valve is gaping and there is no ulceration.[33] In the initial stages, there is mucosal hyperemia, which progresses to erosions and ulcerations. Sloughing of the mucosa with projection of the mucosal remnants may lead to pseudopolyp formation, which can be seen on CT if outlined by air. There is bowel wall thickening, which, however, is less marked as compared with CD (**Fig. 8**). Fistula and abscess formation is also uncommon.[34] Rectal narrowing and increased presacral space are characteristic of UC (**Fig. 9**). The increase in presacral space occurs because of extramural fat proliferation, which has slightly increased attenuation (10–20 Hounsfield units [HU]) compared with normal mesenteric fat (−55 to −75 HU) with intervening areas of soft tissue attenuation.[34] In the chronic stage, the colon has a narrow, ahaustral, and foreshortened appearance (the lead-pipe colon seen on barium studies).[35] The differentiating points of CD and UC are highlighted in **Box 5**.

Inflammation beyond the colonic mucosa and damage to the muscularis propria result in marked colonic dilatation and ahaustral pattern suggestive of toxic megacolon. These findings are more marked in the nondependent loops of bowel like

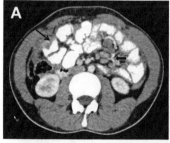
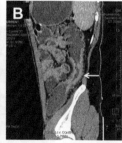
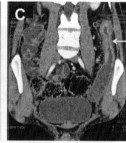

Fig. 5. CECT axial (*A*), CTC sagittal (*B*), and coronal (*C*) images show ileal thickening (*black arrow*), with multiple mesenteric nodes (*block arrow, A*) and descending colon wall thickening (*white arrow; B, C*). Biopsy was suggestive of TB.

Box 4 Differentiation of TB from CD		
Imaging Features	**TB**	**CD**
Stricture	Concentric	Eccentric
Mural stratification	Absent	Present: acute phase Absent: chronic phase
Mesentery	Inflammation	Hyperemia/ vascular engorgement
Lymph nodes	Necrotic rim enhancing	Homogenous mildly enlarged
Fibrofatty proliferation	Less common	More common
Fistula/sinus/abscess	Less common	More common
Enteroliths	Common	Rare
Prestenotic dilatation	Significant	Minimal

Data from Refs.[26–28]

the transverse colon. There is thinning of the colonic wall, nonobstructive dilatation of the colon to at least 6 cm, ascites, and systemic toxicity. It may further be complicated by perforation, pneumatosis, or septic thrombosis.[32,34] The risk of malignancy is high in patients with chronic UC, and regular screening is recommended.

PET WITH FLUDEOXYGLUCOSE F 18/ COMPUTED TOMOGRAPHY IN INFLAMMATORY BOWEL DISEASE

[18]FDG-PET/CT in combination with CTE has been chiefly used in the evaluation of CD. Although [18]FDG-PET alone has been reported to be sensitive and specific in the evaluation of activity in CD,[36] the combination of PET-CTE or PET-CTC increases performance as the bowel is adequately distended.[6,10]

Normally, the small bowel shows diffuse, heterogeneous, and low-level uptake, which is attributed to bowel peristalsis. Closely placed ileal loops in the pelvis may simulate slightly higher or focal uptake, but uptake is less or equal to that of the liver.[37] In disease, the uptake is focal, intense, and higher than that of the liver (**Figs. 10 and 11**).[6] CD may also have a long segment diffuse uptake or show multifocal areas of uptake due to skip involvement. Typical locations of uptake in CD include the terminal ileum with or without involvement of the cecum, jejunum, duodenum, and colon.[9] Ileocecal TB is an important differential diagnosis in endemic areas and is characterized by uptake around the ileocecal junction involving both the ileum and cecum.[16] FDG-PET/CTE also provides information about extramural disease, such as the presence of mesenteric lymphadenopathy, mesenteric fat stranding, mesenteric hyperemia, and sacroiliitis, which would favor IBD. This technique has also been found to be sensitive on detecting fistulae and abscesses in CD. CTE correlation can delineate whether the areas with uptake have abnormal bowel thickening or simply represent undistended or collapsed bowel loops.[6] This correlation adds to the specificity of [18]FDG-PET in delineating disease extent. Quantitative measures of standardized uptake values (SUV) as a measure of disease activity in IBD have been evaluated but were found to be less reproducible as compared with qualitative analysis of uptake. However, in a study by Louis and colleagues,[38] the ratio of SUV over diseased segments and liver correlated significantly with the endoscopic grade of disease.

[18]FDG-PET/CT has a good correlation with endoscopic grade of disease. Although it is 100% sensitive in detecting moderate to severe endoscopic disease (deep ulcers, strictures), it also has good sensitivity (84.4%) in detecting mild to moderate grades of endoscopic inflammation (superficial ulcers).[39] [18]FDG-PET/CT can also detect disease upstream of a stricture, which cannot be negotiated by an endoscope. Thus, it

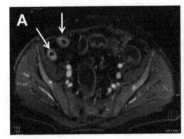
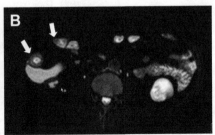

Fig. 6. MR imaging post–gadolinium-enhanced axial image (*A*) shows abnormal enhancement of distal ileal loops (*white arrows*). (*B*) T2-weighted axial image shows wall thickening in distal ileal loops (*block arrows*).

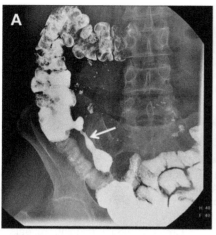
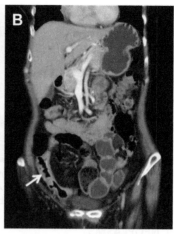

Fig. 7. Barium meal follow through (BMFT) (*A*) and CTE coronal (*B*) images show long segment thickened ileal loop (*white arrow; A, B*) and mesenteric fatty proliferation and mesenteric hyperemia (*black arrow, B*) suggestive of active inflammation in CD.

provides a more global and a noninvasive estimate of disease extent. This capability is especially useful in pediatric patients and in selected adult patients in whom bowel preparation and invasive endoscopy may not be feasible.[40–42] Also in known cases of IBD, it can be useful in monitoring disease activity and response to treatment because of its good correlation with endoscopy. Monitoring response to treatment is important in patients on immunomodulators, such as infliximab, as early nonresponders can be taken off this treatment without subjecting them to the long-term adverse effects of immunosuppressive treatments. [18]FDG-PET/CT provides a more dynamic evaluation of response as compared with morphologic changes, such as bowel thickening, which take a longer time to resolve.[9] Studies have also attempted to differentiate fibrotic strictures from inflammatory strictures in CD as the former requires surgery, whereas the latter can be treated medically. However, this has been less accurate as even fibrotic and mixed strictures show uptake due to a component of associated ongoing inflammation.[39]

[18]FDG/CTC is useful in the follow-up of patients with UC. Das and colleagues[7] performed [18]FDG-PET/CTC in 15 patients with UC and found 98.5% segment-to-segment correlation between disease sites on [18]FDG-PET/CTC and the gold standard colonoscopy. In addition, the disease activity on PET-CTC using the ratio of SUV of disease segment with liver correlated well with the colonoscopic grade of disease. Thus, this technique has the potential to replace colonoscopy as a noninvasive alternative for follow-up in-patients with UC similar to [18]FDG-PET/CTE in CD.

Neutropenic Colitis

Neutropenic enterocolitis is seen in immunosuppressed individuals (leukemia, acquired immunodeficiency syndrome, after transplantation or chemotherapy for malignancy). It usually involves the caecum and ascending colon. CT is the investigation of choice and shows marked circumferential thickening associated with peri-colonic stranding and fluid (**Fig. 12**). It may be complicated by perforation, abscess formation, or hemorrhage.[34]

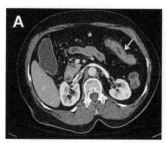
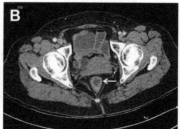
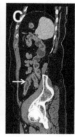

Fig. 8. CTE axial (*A, B*) and sagittal (*C*) images show long segment thickening of descending colon (*arrow, A*) up to rectum (*arrow, B*) also seen on sagittal image (*arrow, C*) with fatty proliferation (*asterisk, A*) suggestive of UC.

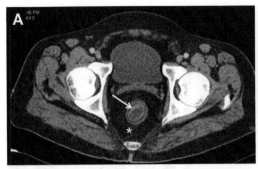
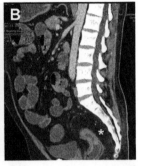

Fig. 9. CTE axial (*A*) and coronal (*B*) images of a patient with UC shows rectal wall thickening with mural stratification and submucosal fatty proliferation (*arrow, A*) suggestive of subacute phase of UC. There is also perirectal fatty proliferation (*asterisk*) also consistent with subacute to chronic phase of UC.

SMALL BOWEL NEOPLASMS

Small bowel neoplasms are rare and usually diagnosed late because of nonspecific clinical presentation. They can present as an annular constricting lesion, mass, or nodule. Neoplasms are characterized by asymmetric focal wall thickening and irregular transition from normal to the involved segment. Usually there is proximal luminal dilatation.[2,43]

Adenocarcinoma is the most common small bowel neoplasm, with carcinoid tumor, lymphoma, and GI stromal tumor being the other primary bowel tumors.[44]

Adenocarcinoma

Adenocarcinoma is the most common primary tumor of small bowel, seen most commonly in the duodenum and proximal jejunum. These may be polypoid, infiltrating or stenosing.[45]

Cross-sectional imaging reveals a well-defined polypoid mass in the duodenum, with central ulceration seen in 10% of cases. Jejunal and ileal lesions are seen as asymmetric wall thickening causing luminal narrowing and bowel obstruction (**Fig. 13**). There is usually annular constriction with proximal shouldering.[46] Heterogeneous enhancement is seen after contrast administration. There may be infiltration of the surrounding fat seen as fat stranding on CT and hyperintensity on T2-weighted fat-suppressed MR sequences.[45]

Carcinoid

Carcinoid is a neuroendocrine tumor seen most commonly in the ileum. It may be seen as an enhancing mucosal polyp, parietal nodule, or focal wall thickening.[2] On triple-phase CT, the mass shows arterial phase enhancement; on MR imaging, it is usually isointense to muscle on

Box 5 Differentiation of CD from UC		
Imaging Features	**CD**	**UC**
Extent of involvement	Segmental skip	Diffuse continuous
Site	Small and large bowel	Colon (rectosigmoid)
Small bowel involvement	Any site	Terminal ileum backwash ileitis
Ileocaecal valve	Stenosed	Open
Symmetry	Asymmetric	Symmetric
Fat proliferation	Mesenteric fat	Perirectal fat
Wall thickness	Marked	Moderate
Mural stratification	Present: acute phase Absent: chronic phase	Present
Wall attenuation	Homogenous: chronic phase	Inhomogenous
Mesenteric hyperemia	Present	Absent
Fistula/sinus/abscess	Common	Rare
Lymph nodes	Usually enlarged	Not enlarged
Toxic megacolon	Less common	More common
Malignant change	Low risk	High risk

Data from Refs.[28,33,34]

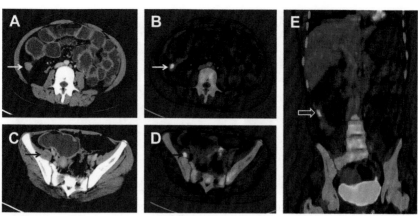

Fig. 10. [18]FDG-PET/CTE images of 18-year-old woman with CD show thickening in ileocecal junction with surrounding fat stranding (*A, white arrow*) and uptake in the corresponding fused [18]FDG-PET/CTE image (*B, white arrow*). Thickening and uptake are also seen at base of cecum (*C, D; black arrow*). Coronal [18]FDG-PET/CTE (*E, open arrow*) images show uptake at ileocecal junction.

T1-weighted images and isointense to mildly hyperintense to muscle on T2-weighted images. Synchronous lesions in the bowel and liver metastases show similar morphology on imaging.[47] Carcinoids are characterized by intense desmoplastic reaction, seen as a spiculated mass in the mesentery (**Fig. 14**), which may show calcification in up to 70% cases.[45]

Non-Hodgkin Lymphoma

Non-Hodgkin lymphoma is the third most common malignancy involving the small bowel. There are 4 main patterns of bowel involvement: diffuse infiltrative form, multiple nodules, mass forming lesion, exophytic masses.[45] Wall thickening associated with lymphoma is usually homogenous and marked. The thickening is in the range of 15 to 20 mm, and the degree of enhancement is lower.[48] This thickening is frequently associated with enlarged lymph nodes (**Fig. 15**).

The pattern of involvement of mesenteric lymph nodes can also help in diagnosing lymphoma. These nodes are homogenous, bulky nodes more commonly involving the margin of the small bowel mesentery. The sandwich sign which is produced by the enlarged lymph nodes in the mesentery encasing the small bowel mesenteric vessels is also commonly seen with lymphoma.[49]

Gastrointestinal Stromal Tumors

Gastrointestinal stromal tumors (GISTs) arise from the interstitial cells of Cajal, within the Auerbach

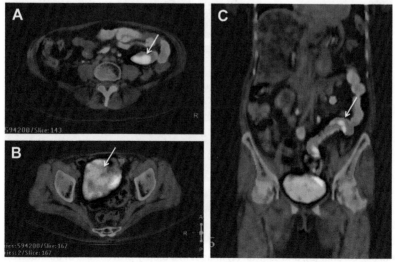

Fig. 11. [18]FDG-PET/CTE images of woman with CD showing [18]FDG uptake in jejunum and ileum on fused PET/CTE image (*white arrows, A–C*).

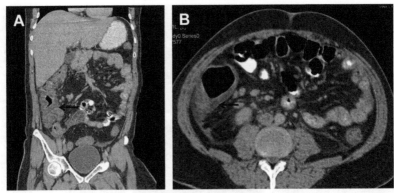

Fig. 12. CT coronal (*A*) and axial (*B*) images of an immunocompromised patient show focal thickening of cecum and ascending colon (*arrows*) consistent with neutropenic colitis.

plexus and can present as submucosal, subserosal/exocentric, or intraluminal masses.[50] Usually these are large masses and can grow exophytically or intraluminally. Histologically, GISTs may be benign, potentially malignant, or malignant. The imaging features favoring malignancy include a diameter greater than 5 cm, irregular shape, internal necrotic component, and heterogeneous contrast enhancement. Distant metastases and locoregional spread are also common with malignant lesions.[2,51]

Metastases

Metastases to the small bowel are infrequent, with melanoma, lung, breast, thyroid, and bowel being

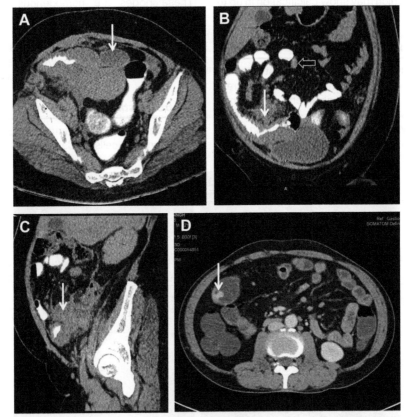

Fig. 13. CECT axial (*A*), coronal (*B*), and sagittal (*C*) images in a biopsy-proven case of adenocarcinoma show focal masslike thickening of distal ileum (*white arrows*) with locoregional lymph node (*block arrow, B*). Axial CT (*D*) image showing polypoid lesion (*white arrow, D*), which can harbor malignancy.

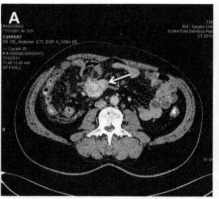
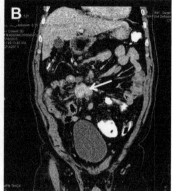

Fig. 14. CECT axial (*A*) and coronal (*B*) images of a proven case of carcinoid show an enhancing mass in mesentery (*white arrow*; *A, B*) and surrounding mesenteric puckering leading to fixed small bowel loops.

the common primary malignancies.[45] They are usually submucosal or subserosal and appear as smooth, round, or polypoid masses with a target appearance. Surface deposits or extramural nodules occur from primary mucinous tumors. These deposits are seen as bowel wall thickening with mesenteric fat stranding.[52]

PET with Fludeoxyglucose F 18/Computed Tomography in Small Bowel Neoplasms

Bowel neoplasms also show increased focal uptake on [18]FDG-PET/CT. Although GISTs show avid focal uptake, lymphomas can present as both focal as well as long segment diffuse uptake.[53] In a setting of CD, long segment involvement can either be due to secondary lymphoma transformation or due to active CD and needs histopathologic correlation.[54] [18]FDG-PET/CT can also detect melanoma metastases, carcinoids, and bowel metastases from unknown primary cancers.[53,55] Location of abnormal sites of uptake can better direct endoscopic biopsies, especially for lesions in small bowel. [68]Gallium (Ga)-labeled

(1, 4, 7, 10-tetraazacyclododecane-1, 4, 7, 10-tetraacetic acid)-1-Nal3-octreotide (^{68}Ga-DOTA-NOC)–PET/CT is used in carcinomas of unknown primary of neuroendocrine origin. Lesions located in the bowel are better appreciated on enterography images, and ^{68}Ga-DOTANOC–PET/CTE has been described as an accurate modality for small bowel carcinoid delineation (**Fig. 16**).[56]

Colonic Carcinoma

Colorectal cancer (CRC) is the third most common malignancy overall in both men and women.[57] Imaging studies help in the staging and preoperative evaluation of the disease. These studies also have a major role to play in the screening and surveillance of CRC.[58]

Carcinoma can be seen as focal or circumferential wall thickening or as a mass on CT. When rectal contrast has been administered, the characteristic annular constricting lesion can be identified. The mass may be heterogeneous with central areas of necrosis. Calcification is occasionally seen in cases of mucinous

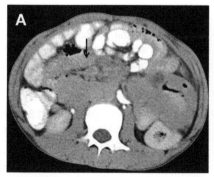
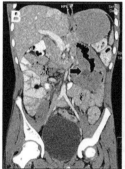
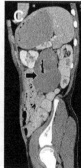

Fig. 15. CECT axial (*A*), coronal (*B*), and sagittal (*C*) images of a proven case of lymphoma show multiple mesenteric lymph nodes (*black arrow, A*) and masslike circumferential thickening and aneurysmal dilatation of proximal jejunum (*block arrows*; *B, C*) suggestive of lymphoma.

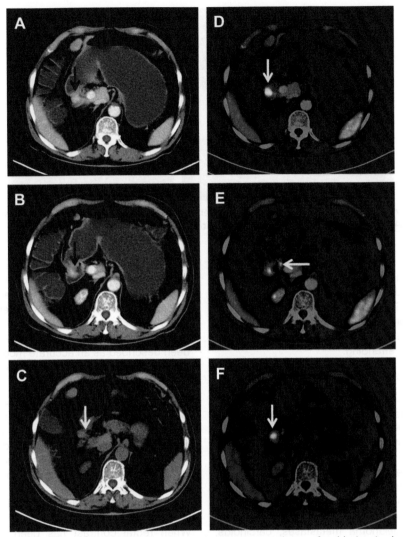

Fig. 16. CTE images in a patient with multiple neuroendocrine tumors show a focal lesion in duodenum (*black arrows*; *A, B*), which was seldom visualized in plain CT image (*white arrow, C*). ^{68}Ga-DOTANOC–PET/CTE images of the same patient show 2 separate lesions with uptake (*white arrow; D, E*). However, PET-CT image without enterography revealed only one lesion (*white arrow, F*). The second lesion (*white arrow, E*) would have been missed in simple PET-CT without enterography.

adenocarcinoma and its metastatic deposits. There can be extension into the perirectal fat seen as soft tissue stranding. Invasion of surrounding structures and fistula formation may be seen in the advanced stages.[57]

Endoluminal images can also be obtained by CTC noninvasively. It allows assessment of the entire mucosal surface, local invasion, vascular anatomy, lymph nodal staging, and the presence of metastases in the abdomen.[59]

On MR imaging, the tumor mass appears isointense to mildly hyperintense (to muscle) on T1-weighted images and hyperintense on T2-weighted images and shows enhancement on the postcontrast scans. T2-weighted images demonstrate the mesorectal fascia better and give more accurate local staging. The use of endorectal coils provides a more precise T stage determination.[57]

PET with Fludeoxyglucose F 18/Computed Tomography Colonography in Screening and Staging of Colorectal Cancers

This technique has also been described for both the detection of colorectal polyps and for staging of patients diagnosed with CRC.[8,60] [18]FDG-PET/CTC has been found to accurately detect and characterize focal adenomatous polyps more than 6 mm in size. In patients diagnosed with CRC, [18]FDG-PET/CTC helps in TNM staging of disease by accurate T staging, detection of metastatic nodes even if subcentimeter in size (N), and detection of distal metastases (M). As compared with gold standard surgical staging, [18]FDG-PET/CTC was about 70% accurate in overall TNM staging and 84% accurate in T staging.[8] Thus, [18]FDG-PET/CTC in CRC can act as a one-stop shop for tumor staging in CRC. [18]FDG-PET/CTC also helps in detecting small synchronous lesions and multiple lesions, especially proximal to an obstruction in case of a non-negotiable colonoscope.[61] [18]FDG-PET/CTC also helps in differentiation from disease recurrence from postoperative fibrosis or scar tissue.[60]

SUMMARY

Cross-sectional imaging plays a pivotal role in the evaluation of the small and large bowel. With the introduction of hybrid PET-CT and PET-MR imaging scanners combining the advantage of anatomic and functional techniques, there has been a paradigm shift in the imaging of various bowel pathologies. In an appropriate clinical setting, judicious use of any of these modalities discussed here can play an important role in clinical decision making.

REFERENCES

1. Markova I, Kluchova K, Zboril R, et al. Small bowel imaging—still a radiologic approach? Biomed Pap Med Fac Univ Palacky Olomouc Czech Repub 2010;154:123–32.
2. Algin O, Evrimler S, Arslan H. Advances in radiologic evaluation of small bowel diseases. J Comput Assist Tomogr 2013;37(6):862–71.
3. Algin O, Evrimler S, Ozmen E, et al. A novel biphasic oral contrast solution for enterographic studies. J Comput Assist Tomogr 2013;37:65–74.
4. Bicik I, Bauerfeind P, Breitbach T, et al. Inflammatory bowel disease activity measured by positron emission tomography. Lancet 1997;350(9073):262.
5. Kresnik E, Gallowitsch HJ, Mikosch P, et al. (18) F-FDG positron emission tomography in the early diagnosis of enterocolitis: preliminary results. Eur J Nucl Med Mol Imaging 2002;29(10):1389–92.
6. Das CJ, Makharia G, Kumar R, et al. PET-CT enteroclysis: a new technique for evaluation of inflammatory diseases of the intestine. Eur J Nucl Med Mol Imaging 2007;34(12):2106–14.
7. Das CJ, Makharia GK, Kumar R, et al. PET/CT colonography: a novel non-invasive technique for assessment of extent and activity of ulcerative colitis. Eur J Nucl Med Mol Imaging 2010;37(4):714–21.
8. Kinner S, Antoch G, Bockisch A, et al. Whole-body PET/CT-colonography: a possible new concept for colorectal cancer staging. Abdom Imaging 2007; 32(5):606–12.
9. Shyn PB. 18F-FDG positron emission tomography: potential utility in the assessment of Crohn's disease. Abdom Imaging 2012;37(3):377–86.
10. Shyn PB, Mortele KJ, Britz-Cunningham SH, et al. Low-dose 18F-FDG PET/CT enterography: improving on CT enterography assessment of patients with Crohn disease. J Nucl Med 2010;51(12): 1841–8.
11. Coakley FV, Gould R, Yeh BM, et al. CT radiation dose: what can you do right now in your practice? AJR Am J Roentgenol 2011;196(3):619–25.
12. Flicek KT, Hara AK, Silva AC, et al. Reducing the radiation dose for CT colonography using adaptive statistical iterative reconstruction: a pilot study. AJR Am J Roentgenol 2010;195(1):126–31.
13. Liu B, Ramalho M, AlObaidy M, et al. Gastrointestinal imaging-practical magnetic resonance imaging approach. World J Radiol 2014;6(8):544–66.
14. Sinha R, Verma R, Verma S, et al. MR enterography of Crohn disease: part 1, rationale, technique, and pitfalls. AJR Am J Roentgenol 2011;197:76–9.
15. Sinha R, Verma R, Verma S, et al. MR enterography of Crohn disease: part 2, imaging and pathologic findings. AJR Am J Roentgenol 2011;197:80–5.
16. Kavaliauskiene G, Ziech ML, Nio CY, et al. Small bowel MRI in adult patients: not just Crohn's disease—a tutorial. Insights Imaging 2011;2:501–13.
17. Gourtsoyannis N, Papanikolaou N, Grammatikakis J, et al. MR enteroclysis protocol optimization: comparison between 3D FLASH with fat saturation after intravenous gadolinium injection and true FISP sequences. Eur Radiol 2001;11:908–13.
18. Deeab DA, Dick E, Sergot AA, et al. Magnetic resonance imaging of the small bowel. Radiography 2011;17:67–71.
19. Prassopoulos P, Papanikolaou N, Grammatikakis J. Rouso- moustakaki M, Maris T, Gourtsoyiannis N. MR enteroclysis imaging of Crohn disease. Radiographics 2001;21(Spec No):S161–72.
20. Fujii T, Naganuma M, Kitazume Y, et al. Advancing magnetic resonance imaging in Crohn's disease. Digestion 2014;89:24–30.
21. Buisson A, Joubert A, Montoriol PF, et al. Diffusion-weighted magnetic resonance imaging for detecting and assessing ileal inflammation in Crohn's disease. Aliment Pharmacol Ther 2013;37:537–45.
22. Oto A, Kayhan A, Williams JTB, et al. Active Crohn's disease in the small bowel: evaluation by diffusion weighted imaging and quantitative dynamic contrast enhanced MR imaging. J Magn Reson Imaging 2011;33:615–24.

23. Kinner S, Hahnemann ML, Forsting M, et al. Magnetic resonance imaging of the bowel: today and tomorrow. Rofo 2015;187:160–7.

24. Fernandes T, Oliveira MI, Castro R, et al. Bowel wall thickening at CT: simplifying the diagnosis. Insights Imaging 2014;5:195–208.

25. Macari M, Megibow AJ, Balthazar EJ. A pattern approach to the abnormal small bowel: observations at MDCT and CT enterography. AJR Am J Roentgenol 2007;188:1344–55.

26. Engin G, Balik E. Imaging findings of intestinal tuberculosis. J Comput Assist Tomogr 2005;29(1): 37–41.

27. Prakash A. Abdominal tuberculosis. In: Gupta AK, Chowdhury V, Khandelwal N, editors. Diagnostic radiology: gastrointestinal and hepatobiliary imaging. 3rd edition. New Delhi (India): Jaypee Brothers; 2009. p. 112–33.

28. Masselli G, Gualdi G. CT and MR enterography in evaluating small bowel diseases: when to use which modality? Abdom Imaging 2013;38:249–59.

29. Soyer P, Boudiaf M, Dray X, et al. CT enteroclysis features of uncomplicated celiac disease: retrospective analysis of 44 patients. Radiology 2009; 253(2):416–24.

30. Masselli G, Gualdi G. MR imaging of the small bowel. Radiology 2012;264(2):333–4.

31. Athanasakos A, Mazioti A, Economopoulos N, et al. Inflammatory bowel disease—the role of cross-sectional imaging techniques in the investigation of the small bowel. Insights Imaging 2015; 6:73–83.

32. Roggeveen MJ, Tismenetsky M, Shapiro R. Ulcerative colitis. Radiographics 2006;26:947–51.

33. Lee SD, Cohen RD. Endoscopy in inflammatory bowel disease. Gastroenterol Clin North Am 2002; 31:119–32.

34. Thoeni RF, Cello JP. CT imaging of colitis. Radiology 2006;240(3):623–38.

35. Carucci LR, Levine MS. Radiographic imaging of inflammatory bowel disease. Gastroenterol Clin North Am 2002;31:93–117.

36. Holtmann MH, Uenzen M, Helisch A, et al. 18F-Fluorodeoxyglucose positron-emission tomography (PET) can be used to assess inflammation noninvasively in Crohn's disease. Dig Dis Sci 2012 Oct;57(10):2658–68.

37. Abouzied MM, Crawford ES, Nabi HA. 18F-FDG imaging: pitfalls and artifacts. J Nucl Med Technol 2005;33(3):145–55 [quiz: 162–3].

38. Louis E, Ancion G, Colard A, et al. Noninvasive assessment of Crohn's disease intestinal lesions with (18)F-FDG PET/CT. J Nucl Med 2007;48(7): 1053–9.

39. Lenze F, Wessling J, Bremer J, et al. Detection and differentiation of inflammatory versus fibromatous Crohn's disease strictures: prospective comparison of 18F-FDG-PET/CT, MR-enteroclysis, and transabdominal ultrasound versus endoscopic/histologic evaluation. Inflamm Bowel Dis 2012;18(12):2252–60.

40. Lemberg DA, Issenman RM, Cawdron R, et al. Positron emission tomography in the investigation of pediatric inflammatory bowel disease. Inflamm Bowel Dis 2005;11(8):733–8.

41. Löffler M, Weckesser M, Franzius C, et al. High diagnostic value of 18F-FDG-PET in pediatric patients with chronic inflammatory bowel disease. Ann N Y Acad Sci 2006;1072:379–85.

42. Skehan SJ, Issenman R, Mernagh J, et al. 18F-fluorodeoxyglucose positron tomography in diagnosis of paediatric inflammatory bowel disease. Lancet 1999;354(9181):836–7.

43. Thulkar S, Gupta AK. Malignant lesions of stomach and small intestine. In: Gupta AK, Chowdhury V, Khandelwal N, editors. Diagnostic radiology: gastrointestinal and hepatobiliary imaging. 3rd edition. New Delhi (India): Jaypee Brothers; 2009. p. 91–111.

44. Amzallag-Bellenger E, Oudjit A, Ruiz A, et al. Effectiveness of MR enterography for the assessment of small-bowel diseases beyond Crohn disease. Radiographics 2012;32:1423–44.

45. Anzidei M, Napoli A, Zini C, et al. Malignant tumours of the small intestine: a review of histopathology, multidetector CT and MRI aspects. Br J Radiol 2011;84(1004):677–90.

46. Sailer J, Zacherl J, Schima W. MDCT of small bowel tumours. Cancer Imaging 2007;7:224–33.

47. Coulier B, Pringot J, Gielen I, et al. Carcinoid tumor of the small intestine: MDCT findings with pathologic correlation. JBR-BTR 2007;90:507–15.

48. Zhu QQ, Zhu WR, Wu JT, et al. Comparative study of intestinal tuberculosis and primary small intestinal lymphoma. World J Gastroenterol 2014;20(15): 4446–52.

49. Dong P, Wang B, Sun QY, et al. Tuberculosis versus non-Hodgkin's lymphomas involving small bowel mesentery: evaluation with contrast-enhanced computed tomography. World J Gastroenterol 2008;14(24):3914–8.

50. Koh JS, Trent J, Chen L. Gastrointestinal stromal tumors: overview of pathologic features, molecular biology, and therapy with imatinib mesylate. Histol Histopathol 2004;19:565–74.

51. Horton KM, Juluru K, Montogomery E, et al. Computed tomography imaging of gastrointestinal stromal tumors with pathology correlation. J Comput Assist Tomogr 2003;28:811–7.

52. Sheth S, Horton KM, Garland MR, et al. Mesenteric neoplasms: CT appearances of primary and secondary tumors and differential diagnosis. Radiographics 2003;23:457–73.

53. Prabhakar HB, Sahani DV, Fischman AJ, et al. Bowel hot spots at PET-CT. Radiographics 2007; 27(1):145–59.

54. Ciarallo A, Makis W, Derbekyan V. Primary peripheral T-cell lymphoma of the colon mimics inflammatory bowel disease: a potential pitfall with F-18 FDG PET/CT imaging. Clinnucl Med 2011;36(7): e61–4.

55. Tatlidil R, Mandelkern M. FDG-PET in the detection of gastrointestinal metastases in melanoma. Melanoma Res 2001;11(3):297–301.

56. Jain TK, Karunanithi S, Dhull VS, et al. Carcinoma of unknown primary of neuroendocrine origin: accurate detection of primary with 68Ga-labelled [1, 4, 7, 10-tetraazacyclododecane-1, 4, 7, 10-tetraacetic acid]-1-Nal3-Octreotide positron emission tomography/computed tomography enterography. Indian J Nucl Med 2014;29(2):122–3.

57. Kalra N, Kang M. Colorectal malignancies. In: Gupta AK, Chowdhury V, Khandelwal N, editors. Diagnostic radiology: gastrointestinal and hepatobiliary imaging. 3rd edition. New Delhi (India): Jaypee Brothers; 2009. p. 154–74.

58. Kekelidze M, D'Errico L, Pansini M, et al. Colorectal cancer: current imaging methods and future perspectives for the diagnosis, staging and therapeutic response evaluation. World J Gastroenterol 2013; 19(46):8502–14.

59. Narayanan S, Kalra N, Bhatia A, et al. Staging of colorectal cancer using contrast-enhanced multidetector computed tomographic colonography. Singapore Med J 2014;55(12):660–6.

60. Veit-Haibach P, Kuehle CA, Beyer T, et al. Diagnostic accuracy of colorectal cancer staging with whole-body PET/CT colonography. JAMA 2006;296(21): 2590–600.

61. Nagata K, Ota Y, Okawa T, et al. PET/CT colonography for the preoperative evaluation of the colon proximal to the obstructive colorectal cancer. Dis Colon Rectum 2008;51(6):882–90.

Diuretic ^{18}F-Fluorodeoxyglucose PET/Computed Tomography in Evaluation of Genitourinary Malignancies

Krishan Kant Agarwal, MD, Shambo Guha Roy, MD, Rakesh Kumar, MD, PhD*

KEYWORDS

- ^{18}F-FDG PET/CT • Diuretics • Urinary bladder cancer • Cervical cancer • Ovarian cancer

KEY POINTS

- The interpretation of fluorodeoxyglucose (FDG) PET/computed tomography (CT) is often challenging for pelvic pathologies because of the physiologic bowel and urinary tract activity.
- Intense radiotracer activity in the urinary tract interferes in image interpretation and leads to false-negative result in diagnosis and detection of local recurrence and regional lymph node metastases.
- It is imperative to minimize unnecessary urinary bladder activity to improve the diagnostic yield of PET/CT.
- Acquiring a postvoid image is simple and time saving, but even small residual urine usually has very high concentration of radioactivity.
- Undistended postvoid bladder leads to poor anatomic delineation thereby limiting urinary bladder wall assessment.

INTRODUCTION

FDG PET scanning is widely used in the evaluation of patients with malignancies.[1] FDG is an analog of glucose in which the hydroxyl group of the second position is replaced by radioactive fluorine (F-18) atom. FDG is taken up by the cells and phosphorylated to FDG-6-phosphate, which does not undergo further metabolism because it is not substrate for glycolysis and remains trapped in the cells.[2] FDG, unlike glucose, cannot be reabsorbed in the proximal tubules of the kidney, and so it is excreted unchanged and gets accumulated in urine.

Accumulation of radiotracer activity in the urinary bladder system may mask the hypermetabolic disease focus and affect the diagnostic accuracy of FDG PET computed tomography (CT). Also, normal physiologic activity in the bowel, endometrium, ovary, and blood vessels may interfere with image interpretation.[3] FDG uptake may vary during different phases of the menstrual cycle.[4] Various benign pathologies also show increased FDG uptake, such as serous and mucinous cystic adenoma, corpus luteal cyst, dermoid cyst, endometriosis, inflammation, pelvic kidney, bladder diverticula, and urinary

The authors have nothing to disclose.

Diagnostic Nuclear Medicine Division, Department of Nuclear Medicine, All India Institute of Medical Sciences, New Delhi 110029, India

* Corresponding author.

E-mail address: rkphulia@yahoo.com

PET Clin 11 (2016) 39–46

http://dx.doi.org/10.1016/j.cpet.2015.07.005

diversions.[5] These physiologic activities are of concern especially in abdominopelvic malignancies, such as cervical, ovarian, endometrial, and bladder cancers.[6–8] It is imperative to be aware of the physiologic uptake of FDG and minimize the unnecessary radioactivity accumulated in the urinary bladder.

VARIOUS TECHNIQUES TO MINIMIZE BLADDER ACTIVITY

There are different methods to minimize bladder activity. The first one is to ask the patient to void just before imaging and acquire imaging caudocranially. This allows imaging of the pelvis before the bladder fills.[9] This is the most commonly applied technique because it simple, easy to follow, and physiologic. However, the problem with this is that even a small volume of residual urine with high FDG concentration can cause masking and therefore difficulty in interpretation of lesions close to the urinary bladder. A second method is use of single-lumen urinary catheter to drain continuously. However, in both scenarios bladder can contain a small amount but highly concentrated radioactive residual urine, which interferes in image interpretation. To avoid this problem a double-lumen Foley catheter can be used. When using a double-lumen catheter normal saline can be injected retrograde into urinary bladder to dilute the radioactive urine. However, bladder irrigation has a few disadvantages, such as increased pain during balloon catheter insertion, pain during urinary bladder irrigation, and increased radiation exposure to the technician performing the irrigation.[10] Even after proper precautions, there is a small chance of introducing infection when inserting a catheter.

Haney and colleagues[11] in their mice study used a double-lumen catheter to empty the undesired activity from urinary bladder. They found that flushing of the bladder provides a substantial attenuation in artifacts, such as streak artifacts. Forty-two percent of the images were spoiled by image artifacts directly attributed to bladder signal before application of the double-lumen catheter. After implementing the double-lumen bladder catheter with flushing, 74% of these images had no bladder signal and 19% of the images had a small bladder signal but no artifacts.

Another reported preparation is use of intravenous diuretic (furosemide), which is a safe and well-tolerated method that enhances urinary flux and allows rapid excretion of the urinary radioactivity. Diuretics used in this purpose enhance renal elimination of the excreted ^{18}F-FDG without interfering with the vesical tumor FDG uptake.

Furosemide is a loop diuretic best suited for this purpose because it causes maximal diuresis, which allows a sufficient time window for reduction of bladder activity, before any significant biologic decay of ^{18}F-FDG has taken place. Urine with a low concentration of ^{18}F-FDG replaced urine with a high concentration of the tracer in the bladder as a result of the diuresis promoted by oral hydration and furosemide.[12]

In our institution, pelvic PET/CT images are obtained using the special technique of forced diuresis using intravenous furosemide (40 mg) in adult patients. Oral fluid intake (around 1.5–2 L) is advised and the patient is asked to void three to four times and then hold urine to allow maximum bladder distention. Pelvic spot view (single bed) PET/CT is then acquired after 1 hour of intravenous furosemide administration. This provides a negative contrast in bladder with nonradioactive urine, which leads to high lesion-to-background ratio. The only problem with this technique is that it is difficult to do in patients who are very sick, have urinary incontinence, or are unconscious and not able to hold urine for more than 15 minutes. In such patients, urinary catheterization is done before FDG tracer injection to minimize radiotracer activity at the pelvic region. It also avoids urinary contamination in such patients.

URINARY BLADDER CANCER

[18]F FDG PET CT has been used in the detection of metastatic spread to regional lymph nodes and distant organs in patients diagnosed with bladder cancer; however, its role in staging is limited. Detection of the primary tumor and local visceral tumor recurrence is limited because of the presence of excreted FDG in the urinary tract, which often masks the urinary bladder lesion and probably the adjacent lymph nodes.[7] An intervention to minimize urinary radioactivity without altering the tumor uptake seems needed because most recurrences of superficial bladder cancer remain confined to the bladder wall (**Figs. 1** and **2**).

Kosuda and colleagues[8] assessed feasibility of bladder cancer imaging with FDG PET. They found that a major pitfall in patients with bladder cancer was intense FDG accumulation in the urine. They minimized the urinary FDG activity by urinary irrigation, but were unable to reduce it to the background level and they found a 40% false-negative rate for detection of recurrent or residual tumor in the bladder.[8]

Koyama and colleagues[10] evaluated the role of ^{18}F FDG PET with continuous bladder irrigation in patients with uterine and ovarian tumors. Continuous urinary bladder irrigation was done manually

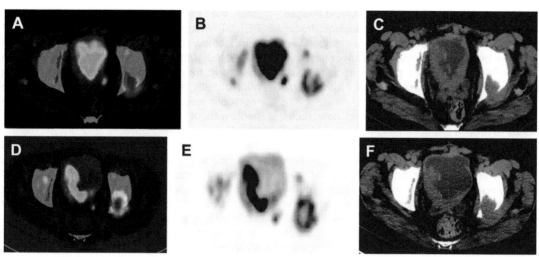

Fig. 1. A 40-year-old man presented with squamous cell carcinoma of urinary bladder. The patient was referred for ¹⁸F-FDG PET/CT scan for staging. In transaxial PET/CT (*A*) and PET (*B*) images, radioactive urine in urinary bladder interferes in image interpretation. Unenhanced axial CT image (*C*) reveals soft tissue thickening involving the entire wall of the bladder. After intravenous diuretic and oral hydration, radiotracer activity from urinary bladder was minimized. Postdiuretic transaxial PET/CT (*D*) and PET (*E*) images showed FDG-avid primary malignant disease in right posterolateral wall of bladder with perivesical lymph node and bilateral pelvic bone metastases corresponding to transaxial CT image (*F*).

using prewarmed physiologic saline solution contained in disposable syringes, beginning 5 minutes before the start of the emission scan and continuing until the end of the scan. The patients were not given any diuretics. In this study, no patients complained of pain during bladder irrigation. In 33 (80%) out of 41 patients, FDG activity in urinary tract was eliminated. However, continuous

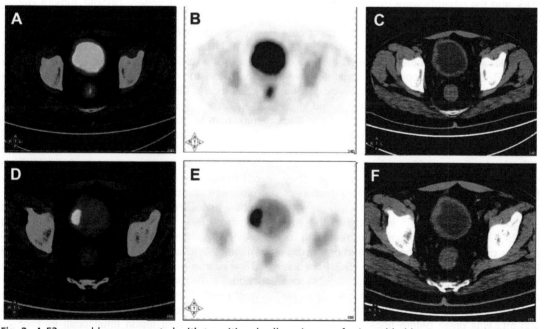

Fig. 2. A 52-year-old man presented with transitional cell carcinoma of urinary bladder. In transaxial PET CT (*A*) and PET (*B*) images, radioactive urine in urinary bladder interferes in image interpretation. In transaxial CT image (*C*), small soft tissue lesion is noted in the right lateral wall of bladder. After intravenous diuretic and oral hydration, radiotracer activity from urinary bladder was minimized with high lesion-to-background ratio. Postdiuretic transaxial PET CT (*D*) and PET (*E*) images showed focal increased FDG tracer uptake in right lateral wall of urinary bladder corresponding to the transaxial CT image (*F*).

bladder irrigation and immediate postvoid images were not effective in reducing physiologic tracer activity in bladder because the kidneys keep filling the bladder with urine with high concentration of ^{18}F-FDG. In eight patients, high residual activities in urinary tract interfere with image interpretation.

Leisure and colleagues[13] studied new techniques to reduce artifact arising from the kidneys, ureters, and bladder using diuretic, intravenous saline infusion, and a bladder catheter. Before FDG PET imaging for pelvis, the urinary catheter was clamped and saline was introduced retrograde into the bladder until full. This technique had many limitations in that it was invasive and retrograde filling of the bladder causes discomfort to the patient. Bladder irrigation also increases radiation to the staff and may cause infection. This technique reduces urinary bladder activity but small amounts of concentrated urine remain that may resemble hypermetabolic lesions, causing even greater difficulty in interpretation.

Kibel and colleagues[14] studied effect of intravenous diuretic during FDG PET/CT in staging of muscle-invasive bladder carcinoma. Foley catheter was placed before injection of FDG, furosemide (20 mg) was administered intravenously approximately 20 minutes after administration of FDG, and the patients were hydrated throughout the study. They found occult metastases in 7 of 42 patients with negative conventional preoperative evaluations.

Drieskens and colleagues[15] studied the role of FDG-PET/CT in the preoperative staging of invasive bladder carcinoma. To increase diagnostic accuracy in detection of primary tumor and local visceral tumor recurrence, such as pelvic and iliac lymph nodes close to areas of high central activity like the bladder, they stimulated urinary flow with 500 mL of saline and 20 mg furosemide intravenously 10 minutes after the FDG injection. They found 90% diagnostic accuracy in detection of local and iliac lymph node metastases.

Anjos and colleagues[12] investigated the role of PET/CT in the detection and restaging of bladder cancer using furosemide and oral hydration to remove the excreted ^{18}F-FDG from the bladder. They did not catheterize urinary bladder before FDG radiotracer injection and also no diuretic was given. Saline infusion (approximately 500 mL) was given before tracer injection. After PET/CT acquisitions, the patients were injected with 20 mg of furosemide intravenously and also oral hydration with 800 to 1000 mL of water. Patients were instructed to void frequently. Additional pelvic images were acquired 1 hour after the intravenous injection of furosemide. PET/CT images before and after furosemide were compared with each other and their findings correlated with MRI, cystoscopy, and biopsy. In this study, they found that PET/CT-delayed image after diuretic and oral hydration revealed hypermetabolic lesions in bladder wall in 6 out of 11 patients without cystectomy and also detected pelvic lymph nodes in two patients and distant metastasis in prostate gland in one patient compared with PET CT done before diuretic. In this study, furosemide was injected at least 2 hours after radiotracer injection, providing excellent urinary radiotracer washout. Bladder activity was reduced to background levels in all bladder-preserved patients. This result could not be obtained in patients with cystectomy because urinary diversions showed higher residual activities. Increased volumetric capacity of bladder diversions led to a slow washout of pooled urinary ^{18}F-FDG and, therefore, larger residual urinary volumes. To overcome this limitation, a higher dose of furosemide and even more delayed images and larger hydration volumes was used. Recurrence is extremely rare in the bladder diversion walls.

Nayak and colleagues[16] studied the effect of diuretic with 1 mg/kg body weight to a maximum of 40 mg of furosemide intravenously in 25 patients with detection of primary tumor and locoregional staging of urinary bladder tumors during FDG PET/CT in our institution. In our study an average dose of 370 MBq of ^{18}F-FDG was injected intravenously. PET/CT acquisition was obtained after a 60-minute uptake period, from the skull base to mid-thigh. After acquisition of the whole-body PET/CT data, all of the patients were injected with 1 mg/kg body weight to a maximum of 40 mg of furosemide intravenously. All patients were asked for 1.5 to 2 L of oral fluid to avoid any dehydration. In addition patients were asked to void two to three times to flush out radioactive urine and then hold urine to allow maximum bladder distention of usually nonradioactive urine. Pelvic PET/CT images were then acquired using the same parameters as detailed previously after 2 hours of whole-body PET/CT imaging. We found that diuretic ^{18}F-FDG PET/CT was true-positive in 24 of 25 (false-negative in one) patients, whereas contrast-enhanced CT was positive in 23 (false-negative in two) patients. In addition, diuretic ^{18}F-FDG PET/CT also detected an extra lesion (multifocal) in 1 of 25 patients. It also demonstrated extravesical infiltration of neighboring structures, such as the urethra, rectovesical fascia, and seminal vesicles. We concluded that diuretic ^{18}F-FDG PET/CT was superior to contrast-enhanced CT in the detection of the primary tumor and locoregional staging (P<.05).

CERVICAL CANCER

Cervical cancer is the third most commonly diagnosed cancer and the fourth leading cause of cancer death in females worldwide.[17] It is preventable and potentially curable if diagnosed early but chances of recurrence are high, varying between 10% and 20% for International Federation of Gynecology and Obstetrics stages IB to IIA and 50% and 70% in locally advanced cases (stages IIB to IVA).[18] Although the International Federation of Gynecology and Obstetrics staging system includes mainly histopathology and clinical examination, imaging modalities are often used for staging and restaging of the disease. ^{18}F-FDG PET detects tumor metabolism and has been proved to be a sensitive tool for lymph node staging and detection of recurrence (**Figs. 3** and **4**).[19,20] FDG PET/CT has also proved to be predictor of survival in patients with cervical cancer.[21,22]

Sugawara and colleagues[23] first tried the feasibility of FDG PET in patients with cervical cancer. They used postvoid images in 11 patients, which substantially reduced the tracer activity in the urinary bladder and improved the visualization of cervical tumors. With this technique, sensitivity in lesion detection was 100%. Postvoid FDG PET scan also improved accuracy for detecting nodal metastases because it minimized excreted radiotracer accumulation in adjoining ureters, which depicts false-negative results in detection of lymph nodal metastases.

Bhoil and colleagues[24] retrospectively analyzed data of 53 patients with recurrent cervical cancer. They found PET/CT to have 90.9% and 87.5% positive and negative predictive value, respectively. They used prehydration of patients with 1000 to 1500 mL of water, but scan was acquired in empty bladder. They took delayed postvoid static pelvic images wherever necessary. For delayed imaging, intravenous furosemide, 40 mg, was also administered to reduce tracer activity in the bladder.

We retrospectively studied the effect of forced diuresis ^{18}F-FDG PET/CT on user interpretability and its incremental value in lesion detection in pelvic malignancies in our institution. After standard whole-body scan, all 51 patients underwent pelvic PET/CT approximately 2 hours after intravenous administration of furosemide and oral hydration. We found that reader interpretability improved in forced-diuresis FDG PET/CT in 78.4% (40 of 51) of studies. The mean interpretability grade improved significantly in the forced-diuresis view (2.90) compared with whole-body scan (1.74; P<.001). Total number of primary tumors identified was increased from 32 to 36 in the postdiuretic view. This increment was seen in bladder carcinoma cases. The forced-diuresis view correctly identified four locally invasive cancers (one bladder, two cervix, one rectum) in which local

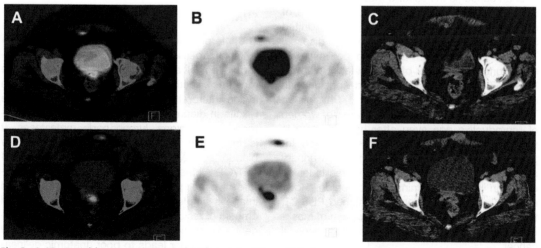

Fig. 3. A 45-year-old woman presented with poorly differentiated squamous cell carcinoma of the cervix. The patient had undergone surgery 2 years ago. The patient was referred for ^{18}F-FDG PET/CT scan for detection of recurrence. In transaxial PET CT (*A*) and PET (*B*) images, increased radiotracer activity in urinary bladder interferes in image interpretation. Transaxial CT image (*C*) revealed hypodense soft tissue thickening in the left vaginal vault. After intravenous diuretic and oral hydration, radiotracer activity from genitourinary tract was decreased. Postdiuretic transaxial PET/CT (*D*) and PET (*E*) images showed left vaginal vault recurrence abutting posterior wall of urinary bladder and deposits involving bilateral rectus muscles corresponding to transaxial CT image (*F*).

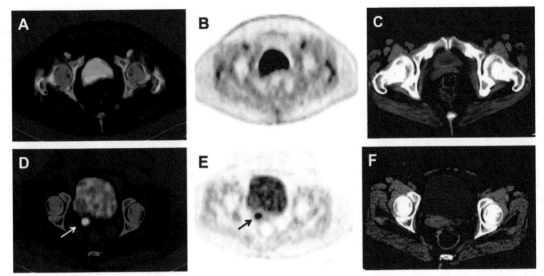

Fig. 4. A 60-year-old woman presented with squamous cell carcinoma of the cervix. The patient was referred for ^{18}F-FDG PET/CT scan for staging. In transaxial PET/CT (*A*) and PET (*B*) images, increased radiotracer activity in urinary bladder interferes in image interpretation. Unenhanced CT image (*C*) revealed small hypodense lesion in cervix. After intravenous diuretic and oral hydration, pelvic spot view (single bed) transaxial PET CT (*D, arrow*) and PET (*E, arrow*) images revealed focal increased FDG tracer uptake in the cervix corresponding to transaxial post-diuretic CT image (*F*).

invasion was missed on whole-body study. In four cases, false-positive suspicious foci disappeared in the forced-diuresis view. SUVmax of bladder decreased significantly after forced diuresis $(19.2 \pm 20.2–1.93 \pm 1.89)$.[25]

OVARIAN CANCER

Ovarian cancer is the second most common genital malignancy in women and leading cause of death from gynecologic cancer in the United States.[26] It usually presents as advance disease. ^{18}F-FDG PET has been shown to be limited in the diagnosis of cancer of the ovaries. However, FDG PET has high sensitivity and specificity in detection of recurrent tumors.[27,28] Physiologic ^{18}F-FDG uptake observed in the ovaries of women of reproductive age even after hysterectomy is reasonably common and may be mistaken for pathologic uptake. FDG tracer uptake in urinary and gastrointestinal tract also interferes in lesion detection in the abdominal/pelvic region. However, with the introduction of combined PET/CT, the interpretation is not as big a problem of masking as in urinary bladder cancer and cervical cancer.

Kamel and colleagues[29] studied the role of forced diuresis in improving the diagnostic accuracy of abdominopelvic ^{18}F-FDG PET. Forced diuretic and oral hydration technique eliminated any significant ^{18}F-FDG activity from the urinary bladder and both ureters in 31 (97%) of 32

patients. In this study during ^{18}F-FDG PET, six indeterminate hot spots that mimicked retroperitoneal lymph node metastases (N = 4), a previously enucleated kidney metastasis (N = 1), and local recurrence of prostate cancer (N = 1) were confined to urinary origin because they disappeared after forced dieresis, so the suspicion of recurrence was confidently ruled out.

SUMMARY

The interpretation of FDG PET/CT is often challenging for pelvic pathologies because of the physiologic bowel and urinary tract activity. Intense radiotracer activity in urinary tract interferes in image interpretation and leads to false-negative results in diagnosis and detection of local recurrence and regional lymph node metastases. It is imperative to minimize unnecessary urinary bladder activity to improve the diagnostic yield of PET/CT. All the techniques described in the literature have their pros and cons. Acquiring a postvoid image is simple and time saving, but even a small amount of residual urine usually has very high concentration of radioactivity. In addition, undistended postvoid bladder leads to poor anatomic delineation thereby limiting urinary bladder wall assessment. Single- or double-lumen catheterization solves this problem but it has to be kept in mind that these are invasive procedures that not only require skill and strict asepsis, and but that are also uncomfortable and even sometimes painful for the patient and carry the chance of infection. Delayed images after forced diuresis with oral hydration give excellent image resolution and have the advantage of imaging the distended bladder with high lesion-to-background contrast. In our experience it is the safest and most convenient method (for patient and physician) that provides excellent image contrast. Urinary catheterization was done in the elderly, children, unconscious, and sick patients before FDG tracer injection to minimize radiotracer activity at the pelvic region. It also avoids urinary contamination in such patients.

REFERENCES

1. Straus LG, Conti PS. The applications of PET in clinical oncology. J Nucl Med 1991;32:623–48.
2. Galagher BM, Fowler JS, Guterson NI, et al. Metabolic traping as a principal of radiopharmaceutical design: some factors responsible for the biodistribution of [18F] 2-deoxy-2-fluoro-D-glucose. J Nucl Med 1978; 19:1154–61.
3. Subhas N, Patel PV, Pannu HK, et al. Imaging of pelvic malignancies with in-line FDG PET-CT: case examples and common pitfalls of FDG PET. Radiographics 2005;25:1031–43.
4. Kim S, Kang KW, Roh JW, et al. Incidental ovarian 18F-FDG accumulation on PET: correlation with the menstrual cycle. Eur J Nucl Med Mol Imaging 2005;32:757–63.
5. Tjalma WA, Carp L, De Beeck BO. False-positive positron emission tomographic scans and computed tomography for recurrent vaginal cancer: pitfalls of modern imaging techniques. Gynecol Oncol 2004; 92:726–8.
6. Harney JW, Wahl RL, Liebert M, et al. Uptake of 2-deoxy-2(18F)fluoro-D-glucosin bladder cancer: animal localization and initial patient positron emission tomography. J Urol 1991;145:279–83.
7. Ahlstrom H, Malmstrom PU, Letocha H, et al. Positron emission tomography in the diagnosis and staging of urinary bladder cancer. Acta Radiol 1996;37: 180–5.
8. Kosuda S, Kison PV, Grenough R, et al. Preliminary assessment of fluorine-18 fluorodeoxyglucose positron emission tomography in patients with bladder cancer. Eur J Nucl Med 1997;24:615–20.
9. Nakamoto Y, Saga T, Fujii S. Positron emission tomography application for gynecologic tumors. Int J Gynecol Cancer 2005;15(5):701–9.
10. Koyama K, Okamura T, Kawabe J, et al. Evaluation of 18F-FDG PET with bladder irrigation in patients with uterine and ovarian tumors. J Nucl Med 2003; 44:353–8.
11. Haney CR, Parasca AD, Ichikawa K, et al. Reduction of image artifacts in mice by bladder flushing with a novel double-lumen urethral catheter. Mol Imaging 2006;5:175–9.
12. Anjos DA, Etchebehere EC, Ramos CD, et al. 18F-FDG PET/CT delayed images after diuretic for restaging invasive bladder cancer. J Nucl Med 2007; 48:764–70.
13. Leisure GP, Vesselle HJ, Faulhaber PF, et al. Technical improvements in fluorine-18-FDG PET imaging of the abdomen and pelvis. J Nucl Med Technol 1997;25:115–9.
14. Kibel AS, Dehdashti F, Katz MD, et al. Prospective study of [18F]fluorodeoxyglucose positron emission tomography/computed tomography for staging of muscle-invasive bladder carcinoma. J Clin Oncol 2009;27:4314–20.
15. Drieskens O, Oyen R, Van Poppel H, et al. FDG-PET for preoperative staging of bladder cancer. Eur J Nucl Med Mol Imaging 2005;32:1412–7.
16. Nayak B, Dogra PN, Naswa N, et al. Diuretic 18F-FDG PET/CT imaging for detection and locoregional staging of urinary bladder cancer: prospective evaluation of a novel technique. Eur J Nucl Med Mol Imaging 2013;40:386–93.
17. Jemal A, Bray F, Center MM, et al. Global cancer statistics. CA Cancer J Clin 2011;61:69–90.
18. Waggoner SE. Cervical cancer. Lancet 2003;361: 2217–25.
19. Leblanc E, Gauthier H, Querleu D, et al. Accuracy of 18-fluoro-2-deoxy-D-glucose positron emission tomography in the pretherapeutic detection of occult para-aortic node involvement in patients with a locally advanced cervical carcinoma. Ann Surg Oncol 2011;18:2302–9.
20. Xiao Y, Wei J, Zhang Y, et al. Positron emission tomography alone, positron emission tomography-computed tomography and computed tomography in diagnosing recurrent cervical carcinoma: a systematic review and meta-analysis. Arch Med Sci 2014;10:222–31.
21. Schwarz JK, Siegel BA, Dehdashti F, et al. Association of posttherapy positron emission tomography with tumor response and survival in cervical carcinoma. JAMA 2007;298:2289–95.
22. Dhull VS, Sharma P, Sharma DN, et al. Prospective evaluation of 18F-fluorodeoxyglucose positron emission tomography-computed tomography for response evaluation in recurrent carcinoma cervix: does metabolic response predict survival? Int J Gynecol Cancer 2014;24:312–20.
23. Sugawara Y, Eisbruch A, Kosuda S, et al. Evaluation of FDG PET in patients with cervical cancer. J Nucl Med 1999;40:1125–31.
24. Bhoil A, Mittal BR, Bhattacharya A, et al. Role of F-18 fluorodeoxyglucose positron emission tomography/computed tomography in the detection of recurrence in patients with cervical cancer. Indian J Nucl Med 2013;28:216–20.

25. Kumar K, Singh H, Soundararajan R, et al. Forced diuresis 18F-FDG PET-CT in pelvic malignancies: incremental value and effect on reader interpretability. Eur J Nucl Med Mol Imaging 2014;41(Suppl 2): S151–705.

26. Jemal A, Murray T, Ward E, et al. Cancer statistics, 2005. CA Cancer J Clin 2005;55(1):10–30 [Erratum appears in CA Cancer J Clin 2005;55:259].

27. Pandit-Taskar N. Oncologic imaging in gynecologic malignancies. J Nucl Med 2005;46:1842–50.

28. Kumar R, Alavi A. PET imaging in gynecologic malignancies. Radiol Clin North Am 2004;42:1155–67.

29. Kamel EM, Jichlinski P, Prior JO, et al. Forced diuresis improves the diagnostic accuracy of 18F-FDG PET in abdominopelvic malignancies. J Nucl Med 2006;47:1803–7.

Role of PET/Computed Tomography in Radiofrequency Ablation for Malignant Pulmonary Tumors

CrossMark

Mitsunori Higuchi, MD, PhD*, Hiroyuki Suzuki, MD, PhD,
Mitsukazu Gotoh, MD, PhD

KEYWORDS

- 18-Fluorodeoxyglucose PET • Computed tomography • Radiofrequency ablation
- Thoracic malignancies

KEY POINTS

- Radiofrequency ablation (RFA) is one of the interventional radiological techniques for pulmonary malignancies.
- Currently, the complication rates after RFA are high, even though the grade of adverse events is low.
- 18F fluorodeoxyglucose PET (FDG-PET) is a useful tool for evaluating the therapeutic effects of RFA.
- Early-phased FDG-PET after RFA shows FDG uptake because of the local inflammatory changes.
- FDG-PET at 3 to 6 months after RFA is important for predicting local recurrence.

INTRODUCTION

Surgical resection has played the main role in the local control of various malignancies; however, comorbidity prevents some patients from undergoing definitive surgery. Microwave ablation or radiofrequency ablation (RFA) are local ablative procedures in which thermal or heat energy is used and tissues are destroyed by thermocoagulation. RFA of neoplastic lesions is gaining popularity in clinical practice because of its minimally invasive nature. RFA was reported for the first time in 2000.[1] Since then, several studies have provided indirect evidence that RFA improves survival.[2–5] RFA is a promising alternative to both surgery and radiotherapy for tumor elimination in patients with primary or metastatic liver neoplasms or other malignancies of the lungs, kidneys, pancreas, thyroid, bone, and soft tissues. The technical success of cancer surgery can be evaluated by pathologic examination of the resected specimens, but nonsurgical procedures need various imaging techniques to verify their adequacy and completeness. Contrast-enhanced computed tomography (CT) and MR imaging have been used to assess the staging and follow-up of various malignancies before and after treatment.[6–8] However, changes at the tissue level in response to the ablative procedure hamper the use of CT and MR imaging to detect or rule out residual disease after ablation. The combination of 18F fluorodeoxyglucose PET (FDG-PET) and CT is an effective tool for assessing treatment response and surveillance of disease recurrence. Many investigators have reported the utility of FDG-PET in evaluating therapeutic response prospectively or retrospectively.[9–12] Complete disappearance of FDG-PET accumulation is an indicator of a low probability of local recurrence and better prognosis after treatment such as surgery, radiation, chemotherapy, and

The authors have nothing to disclose.
Chest Surgery, School of Medicine, Fukushima Medical University, 1-Hikarigaoka, Fukushima 960-1295, Japan
* Corresponding author.
E-mail address: higuchi@fmu.ac.jp

PET Clin 11 (2016) 47–55
http://dx.doi.org/10.1016/j.cpet.2015.08.002
1556-8598/16/$ – see front matter © 2016 Elsevier Inc. All rights reserved.

RFA. In this article, the role of PET/CT after RFA is highlighted and the following topics are discussed: (1) indications for RFA, (2) RFA technique and expected complications, (3) prognosis after RFA, (4) imaging protocol, (5) imaging findings, (6) imaging comparison between FDG-PET and CT scan, (7) optimal follow-up schedule, (8) evaluation of recurrence, (9) pitfalls, and (10) future directions.

CLINICAL BACKGROUND
Non–Small Cell Lung Cancer

Lung cancer is the leading cause of cancer-related death worldwide.[13] Non–small cell lung cancer (NSCLC) constitutes approximately 80% of primary malignant tumors in the lung.[14] Compared with nonsurgical therapy, surgical resection of NSCLC in patients without metastases to other organs can achieve improved long-term survival. However, only approximately one-third of patients are eligible for surgery, and most patients have widespread disease at the time of diagnosis. Additionally, given the increased age of many populations, comorbidity that makes patients poor surgical candidates is increasingly common.[15] Patients with early-stage disease who are medically unfit for surgery, but who have sufficient pulmonary function, might be candidates for radiotherapy with curative intent. Previous reports show that patients ineligible for surgery who were treated with definitive radiotherapy achieved a 5-year survival of 10% to 27%.[16,17] Recently, stereotactic body radiotherapy has caused a paradigm shift in treatment of inoperative patients with early-stage NSCLC.[18,19]

Metastatic Lung Tumor

The lung is the second most frequent site of metastatic diseases. Many series have documented survival benefits of surgical resection in selected patients with pulmonary metastases of favorable histology, especially colorectal carcinoma. However, only a few patients are suitable candidates for resection because of an associated extrapulmonary disease, the extent and location of lesions in the lung, or concurrent medical conditions. Moreover, the high risk of recurrence and the need to remove functioning lung tissue along with the lesions restricts surgical indications.[20]

Other Pulmonary Malignant Tumors

In addition to primary lung cancer and metastatic pulmonary malignancies, there are various other types of malignant pulmonary tumors, which include bronchial gland carcinoma, neuroendocrine tumor, and lymphoma.

INDICATIONS FOR RADIOFREQUENCY ABLATION OF PULMONARY MALIGNANT TUMORS

In general, RFA is used to treat primary and metastatic lung malignancies. In patients with primary NSCLC or metastatic lung tumor, who are not surgical candidates because of poor cardiopulmonary reserve, and in those with poor lung function that precludes external beam radiotherapy, or those who refuse surgery or irradiation, RFA is an effective treatment option. The criteria for general unresectability of pulmonary malignancies are shown in **Table 1**. However, there are some limitations to the indications for RFA, such as the tumors being adjacent to pulmonary vessels or bronchi larger than 5 mm in diameter, or subpleural lesions. The best tumor size for RFA is 4 cm or smaller in diameter, and the number of tumors is not a contraindication. Prior pneumonectomy is also not necessarily a contraindication to RFA in the remaining lung. Pulmonary function is also a definitive criterion for RFA because there is a risk of exacerbation of chronic obstructive pulmonary disease or interstitial pneumonia after RFA. Exclusion criteria include cardiac pacemakers and implantable cardioverter defibrillators, evidence of bleeding, abnormal blood coagulation laboratory values, pregnancy, and infection. The indications and contraindications for RFA of pulmonary malignancies are described in **Table 2**.

Table 1 Criteria of unresectability for pulmonary malignancies	
Major criteria:	Predictive postoperative (ppo) FEV1.0% $\leq$60% ppo DLCO $\leq$50%
Minor criteria:	ppo FEV1.0% $\leq$50% ppo DLCO $\leq$60% Pulmonary arterial pressure >40 mm Hg on echocardiography Left ventricular ejection fraction $\leq$40% PS3 or PS4 PaO$_2$ at rest $\leq$55 mm Hg or SpO$_2$ on room air $\leq$88%

Unresectability is determined for patients with at least 1 major or 2 minor criteria.
Abbreviations: DLCO, diffusing capacity of the lungs for carbon monoxide; FEV1, forced expiratory volume in 1 second; PaO$_2$, partial pressure of oxygen in arterial blood; PS, performance status; SpO$_2$, peripheral capillary oxygen saturation.

Table 2
Inclusion and exclusion criteria of radiofrequency ablation

Inclusion criteria:	ECOG performance status ≤2 Tumor size <40 mm and located in the periphery of the lung Measurable disease as defined by RECIST
Exclusion criteria:	Pacemaker or ICD implantation Evidence of bleeding diathesis or abnormal blood coagulation laboratory values Pregnancy Infection

Abbreviations: ECOG, Eastern Cooperative Oncology Group; ICD, implantable cardioverter defibrillator; RECIST, Response Evaluation Criteria in Solid Tumors.

RADIOFREQUENCY ABLATION TECHNIQUE AND EXPECTED COMPLICATIONS

RFA procedures are performed in patients using local infiltration of lidocaine for anesthesia, and if necessary, administration of fentanyl or midazolam for analgesia. An electrode is percutaneously inserted under ultrasonography or CT guidance. The electrode is introduced into the tumor and is connected to an RF generator (**Fig. 1**). The initial power applied is 20 W, which is subsequently increased until roll-off is achieved (sharply decreased power output owing to increasing tissue impedance from coagulation). Electric current passes from the active RFA electrode through the tissue, causing ion agitation and cellular heating that induces immediate and anaplastic cellular damage, leading to coagulation necrosis.[21] Blood pressure, oxygen levels, and electrocardiography activity are monitored during the procedure.

Occasionally, RFA is associated with immediate or delayed complications in the ablation zone. Infection and abscess formation are some of the major complications of this procedure. Ablation of pulmonary lesions is sometimes associated with pleural effusion, pneumothorax, hemorrhage, and infection. Some reports show a morbidity rate of 50% to 70%; comprising mostly grade 1 or 2 adverse effects, scored according to the National Cancer Institute Common Terminology Criteria for Adverse Events version 4.0.[22] Procedural mortality rate is less than 1%. Complications such as infection and abscess formation can persistently concentrate FDG. Therefore, familiarity with the clinical signs and symptoms of abscess, such as persistent pain and fever is also most important.

PROGNOSIS AFTER RADIOFREQUENCY ABLATION FOR PULMONARY MALIGNANCIES

The overall local control rate for primary lung cancer and pulmonary metastasis after RFA is 70% to 76% at 2 years.[9,23] In other words, 24% to 30% of malignant pulmonary tumors recur locally within 2 years after RFA. However, even if the tumors recur as local lesions, repeated RFA can be performed on a case-by-case basis. Overall 2-year survival rates are 48% to 84%.[9,24] If these results are restricted to cancer-specific survival, 2-year overall survival rates are improved to more than 73%. A previous prospective study showed that patients with stage I NSCLC had a 2-year overall survival rate of 75% (45%–92%) and a 2-year cancer-specific survival of 92% (66%–99%).[24]

IMAGING PROTOCOL

FDG-PET provides information on tumor localization and growth based on increased metabolism and glucose uptake of malignant cells. Before PET, all patients fast for at least 6 hours. Blood glucose concentration is checked before PET. Patients receive an intravenous injection of 3.7 MBq/kg 18F-FDG. After 1 hour of rest, whole-body PET images are acquired. Using CT images for guidance, a region of interest is drawn over the target tumors. Maximum standardized uptake value (SUVmax) is calculated for each tumor.

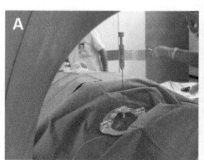 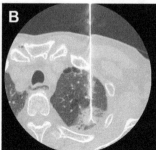

Fig. 1. A Le Veen needle with 10 retractable hooks, with a maximum diameter of 2 to 4 cm, was percutaneously inserted under CT guidance (*A*). Intraoperative CT image shows adequate insertion of the needle into the target tumor (*B*). The initial power applied was 20 W, which was subsequently increased until roll-off (sharply decreased power output owing to increasing tissue impedance from coagulation) was achieved.

IMAGING FINDINGS

Glucose uptake in most normal cell types is regulated by insulin level, whereas in malignant cells, glucose and FDG is taken up predominantly through the Glut-1 transporter, which is independent of the presence of insulin. Thus, FDG-PET allows a whole-body survey, showing metabolic activity of malignant tissues, thereby providing substantial additional information to conventional anatomic imaging. In general, the tumor size on CT before RFA is an important factor in predicting local control of lung tumors after RFA.[25–28] However, the mass size after RFA is not a reliable factor. When malignant cells are destroyed by thermocoagulation, the cells in the ablated area do not concentrate FDG after complete ablation of the tumor. The lack of FDG uptake is reflected as a photopenic area on the FDG-PET image obtained 7 days after RFA (**Fig. 2**), whereas the mass in the original region remains on CT (**Fig. 3**). This is one of the pitfalls when evaluating the ablated area by FDG-PET, which is described in the next section.

IMAGING COMPARISON BETWEEN FLUORODEOXYGLUCOSE-PET AND COMPUTED TOMOGRAPHY SCAN

FDG-PET can evaluate viable cells and it is more sensitive than CT for detection of solitary primary lung tumors.[29,30] A previous prospective analysis showed that FDG-PET/CT had 96% sensitivity and 82% to 88% specificity when compared with sensitivity and specificity of 96% and 53% of CT.[29,31] In identification of pulmonary tumor, FDG-PET is considered to be superior to clinical and morphologic criteria.[32] FDG-PET is accurate in differentiating benign from malignant lesions as small as 1 cm,[33] and overall sensitivity of 96% (range, 83%–100%), specificity of 79% (range, 52%–100%), and accuracy of 91% (range, 86%–100%) can be expected.[34–36] We previously showed the usefulness of SUVmax for the prognosis of patients with pathologic stage I lung adenocarcinoma. In the article, we calculated SUVmax cutoff value as 2.5 according to receiver operating characteristic curve, and also showed that disease-free survival after surgery less than 2.5 of SUVmax was significantly better compared with the patients more than 2.5 of SUVmax.[37]

These results are dependent on SUVmax cutoff values, which each institution decides individually, and there is no universal value. To resolve this problem, Shiono and colleagues[38] demonstrated a corrected SUV, which they termed the SUV index, and calculated this as the ratio of tumor SUV(max) to liver SUV(mean). This SUV index is reproducible and is a significant predictor of NSCLC recurrence. Many investigators have also reported the utility of FDG-PET in evaluating therapeutic response prospectively or retrospectively.[9–11] A general shortcoming of follow-up with CT alone is the existence of the postablation mass that consists of the original lesion and surrounding normal lung.[39] Response criteria fail in this situation because they rely on size[40] in a situation in which the postablation mass is almost always larger than the original lesion (**Fig. 4**). Therefore, imaging with combined 18F-FDG-PET/CT offers many advantages over diagnostic CT alone in the pre- and post-RFA assessment of malignant pulmonary lesions. Complete disappearance of FDG accumulation is an indicator of a low probability of local recurrence and better

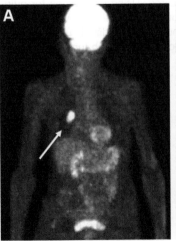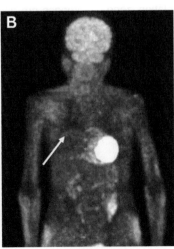

Fig. 2. An 80-year-old woman without previous malignancies was diagnosed with pulmonary adenocarcinoma, 2.5 cm in diameter, in right S6 segment. Her PET image before RFA was SUVmax 11.5 (*arrow*) (*A*) and there was little accumulation of FDG in this main tumor 7 days after RFA (*arrow*) (*B*).

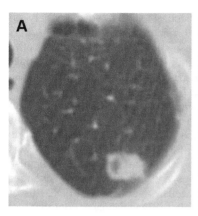
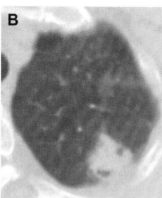

Fig. 3. A 76-year-old man with 1.0 cm-diameter recurrent tumor in left S1+2 segment before RFA (*A*). The mass in the original region 7 days after RFA remained and was larger than the original lesion on CT scan, which provided no information about the viability of this mass (*B*).

prognosis after treatment such as surgery, radiation therapy, and chemotherapy in patients with lung cancer.[41–45]

OPTIMAL FOLLOW-UP SCHEDULE WITH FLUORODEOXYGLUCOSE-PET

The optimal follow-up schedule for FDG-PET is still controversial. A recent prospective study showed the usefulness of FDG-PET as an evaluation tool after RFA, and described the optimal follow-up schedule with FDG-PET.[9] This study demonstrated that FDG accumulation is decreased in successfully treated pulmonary tumor by 3 to 6 months after RFA, and that the SUVmax in cases of local recurrence at 3 to 6 months after RFA is significantly higher than that in successfully ablated tumors.[9] A retrospective study also

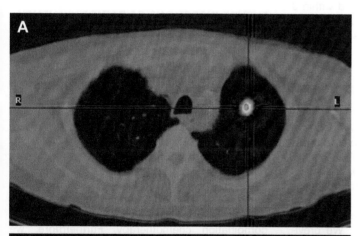
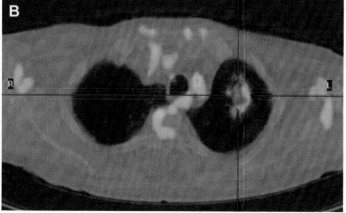

Fig. 4. A 78-year-old man with recurrent tumor in left S1+2 segment before RFA had an SUVmax of 17.7 (*A*). During the chronic phase 4 weeks after RFA, the accumulation of the inner zone decreased and that of the outer zone was unchanged (SUVmax 2.9) (*B*).

showed that FDG-PET at 3 to 6 months after RFA is important for predicting recurrence.[11] Other reports show the usefulness of FDG-PET during the early periods after RFA,[46] and that FDG-PET at 4 or more weeks after RFA is useful in an animal lung model.[28] However, FDG-PET at 3 to 6 months after RFA is more reasonable for the following reason. Immediately after RFA, the ablated tumor consists of an inner zone and an outer zone. Coagulation necrosis is observed in the inner zone, and the outer zone shows congestion. In the subacute phase at 1 week after RFA, the necrotic area of the inner zone shows progression, and the outer zone shows inflammatory change, including infiltration of neutrophils, lymphocytes, and macrophages. During the chronic phase at 4 to 8 weeks after RFA, the size of the inner zone decreases and the outer zone of the inflammatory granulation tissue undergoes fibrous transformation. The outer zone of granulation tissue persists until 3 months after RFA, and this results in the accumulation of FDG, which is false positive (see **Fig. 4**). According to some valuable reports, the following schedule is optimal: FDG-PET and CT are performed at 7 to 14 days after RFA. These imaging evaluations are also performed within 3 to 6 months after RFA and patients are followed by FDG-PET and CT every 3 months for 2 years (**Fig. 5**).

EVALUATION OF RECURRENCE AFTER RADIOFREQUENCY ABLATION

Metabolic imaging can enhance evaluation of ablated lesions and obviate sole reliance on parameters such as size and contrast enhancement. Early detection of recurrence after ablation is critical because there is an opportunity to repeat the ablation as salvage for recurrence. Successful repeated ablation is best performed on small recurrences rather than large ones.[25] We previously demonstrated that FDG accumulation is

decreased in successfully treated pulmonary tumors by 3 to 6 months after RFA. The SUVmax in cases of local recurrence at 3 to 6 months after RFA is significantly higher than that in successfully ablated tumors, although the SUVmax values in both groups at 7 to 14 days after RFA do not differ significantly (**Fig. 6**).[9] If the SUVmax at 3 to 6 months after RFA is increasing again, it indicates local recurrence (**Fig. 7**). Other previous reports show that FDG-PET at 3 to 6 months after RFA is important for predicting recurrence.[10,11] Because of these findings and the inflammatory changes mentioned previously, a schedule of FDG-PET at 3 to 6 months after RFA is widely accepted.

PITFALLS

When a lung lesion undergoes ablation, a central zone of coagulation necrosis is formed that is surrounded by an outer zone of congestion, which, within a few days, shows inflammatory changes caused by the recruitment of neutrophils, lymphocytes, and macrophages.[28,47] Hence, the periphery of the necrotic zone shows increased FDG uptake for a few days when PET is used for RFA evaluation.

FUTURE DIRECTIONS OF RADIOFREQUENCY ABLATION AND RADIOGRAPHIC IMPROVEMENT FOR PULMONARY MALIGNANCIES

RFA is one of the interventional radiological techniques for pulmonary malignancies. The procedure is similar to CT-guided lung biopsy and therefore it is a commonly applied technique. Currently, the complication rates after RFA are high, even though the grade of adverse events is low. Technical and mechanical improvements to reduce the incidence of adverse events are expected. This procedure can improve patient outcomes with conventional radiotherapy or combination chemotherapy. Furthermore, we have no data for long-term outcome of patients

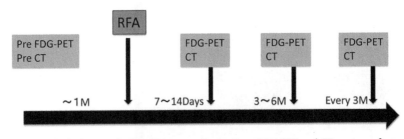

Fig. 5. Follow-up schedule before and after RFA at our institution. FDG-PET and CT were performed before and 7 to 14 days after RFA. Imaging evaluation was also performed within 3 to 6 months after RFA, and patients were followed by FDG-PET and CT every 3 months for 2 years.

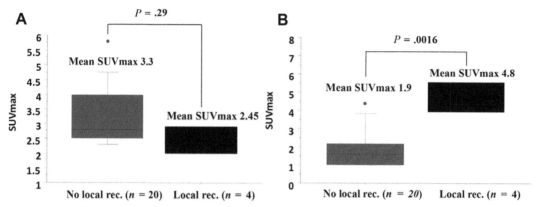

Fig. 6. Comparison of SUVmax between cases with and without local recurrence at 7 to 14 days after RFA (*A*) and 3 to 6 months after RFA (*B*). FDG-PET at 3 to 6 months after RFA is significantly correlated with local recurrence. rec., recurrence.

after RFA; therefore, the accumulation of each patient's data collected from collaborating institutions, or a multicenter prospective study that evaluates the long-term prognosis after RFA is needed to acquire new medical evidence.

ACKNOWLEDGMENTS

The following individuals also contributed to this article as coauthors: Hironori Takagi, MD, Yuki Owada, MD, Takuya Inoue, MD, Yuzuru Watanabe, MD, Mitsuro Fukuhara, MD, Takumi

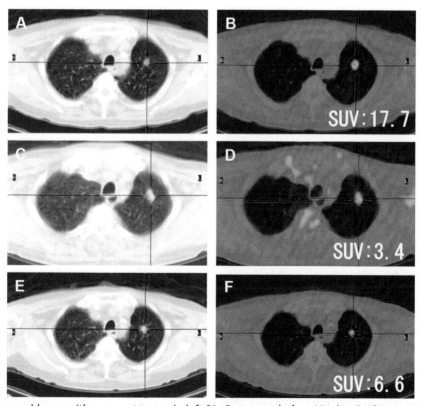

Fig. 7. A 78-year-old man with recurrent tumor in left S1+2 segment before RFA (*A, B*). This case is the same as that described in **Fig. 4**. FDG-PET 2 months after RFA showed remnant FDG accumulation in the lesion (*C, D*), although SUVmax value decreased to 3.4. In the PET image at 6 months after RFA (*E, F*), the SUVmax value increased again and this case was diagnosed with local recurrence by transbronchial lung biopsy, even though the tumor mass on CT scan decreased compared with the CT image before RFA (*A, E*).

Yamaura, MD, Satoshi Muto, MD, Naoyuki Okabe, MD, PhD, Yuki Matsumura, MD, Takeo Hasegawa, MD, PhD, Atsushi Yonechi, MD, PhD, Jun Osugi, MD, PhD, Mika Hoshino, MD, PhD, and Yutaka Shio, MD, PhD.

REFERENCES

1. Dupuy DE, Zagoria RJ, Akerley W, et al. Percutaneous radiofrequency ablation of malignancies in the lung. AJR Am J Roentgenol 2000;174:57–9.

2. Lencioni RA, Allgaier HP, Cioni D, et al. Small hepatocellular carcinoma in cirrhosis: randomized comparison of radiofrequency thermal ablation versus percutaneous ethanol injection. Radiology 2003; 228:235–40.

3. Lin SM, Lin CJ, Lin CC, et al. Radiofrequency ablation improves prognosis compared with ethanol injection for hepatocellular carcinoma < or = 4cm. Gastroenterology 2004;127:1714–23.

4. Shiina S, Teratani T, Obi S, et al. A randomized controlled trial of radiofrequency ablation with ethanol injection for small hepatocellular carcinoma. Gastroenterology 2005;129:122–30.

5. Siperstein AE, Berber E, Ballem N, et al. Survival after radiofrequency ablation of colorectal liver metastases: 10-year experience. Ann Surg 2007;246: 559–65.

6. Schima W, Kulinna C, Langenberger H, et al. Liver metastases of colorectal cancer: US, CT or MR? Cancer Imaging 2005;5:S149–56.

7. Bipat S, van Leeuwen MS, Comans EF, et al. Colorectal liver metastases: CT, MR imaging, and PET for diagnosis—meta-analysis. Radiology 2005;237: 123–31.

8. Quaia E, D'Onofrio M, Palumbo A, et al. Comparison of contrast-enhanced ultrasonography versus baseline ultrasound and contrast-enhanced computed tomography in metastatic disease of the liver: diagnostic performance and confidence. Eur Radiol 2006;16:1599–609.

9. Higuchi M, Honjo H, Shigihara T, et al. A phase II study of radiofrequency ablation therapy for thoracic malignancies with evaluation by FDG-PET. J Cancer Res Clin Oncol 2014;140:1957–63.

10. Alafate A, Shinya T, Okumura Y, et al. The maximum standardized uptake value is more reliable than size measurement in early follow-up to evaluate potential pulmonary malignancies following radiofrequency ablation. Acta Med Okayama 2013;67:105–12.

11. Higaki F, Okumura Y, Sato S, et al. Preliminary retrospective investigation of FDG-PET/CT timing in follow-up of ablated lung tumor. Ann Nucl Med 2008;22:157–63.

12. Weber WA. Use of PET for monitoring cancer therapy and for predicting outcome. J Nucl Med 2005; 46:983–95.

13. Surveillance, Epidemiology, and End Results (SEER) Cancer Statistics Review, 1975–2010. Available at: http://seer.cancer.gov/csr/1975_2010. Accessed June 14, 2013.

14. Hoffman PC, Mauer AM, Vokes EE. Lung cancer. Lancet 2000;355:479–85.

15. Silvestri GA, Sherman C, Williams T, et al. Caring for the dying patient with lung cancer. Chest 2001;122: 1028–36.

16. Dosoretz DE, Katin MJ, Blitzer PH, et al. Radiation therapy in the management of medically inoperable carcinoma of the lung: results and implications for future treatment strategies. Int J Radiat Oncol Biol Phys 1992;24:309.

17. Gauden S, Ramsay J, Tripcony L. The curative treatment by radiotherapy alone of stage I non-small cell carcinoma of the lung. Chest 1995;108:1278–82.

18. Guckenberger M, Allgäuer M, Appold S, et al. Safety and efficacy of stereotactic body radiotherapy for stage I non-small-cell lung cancer in routine clinical practice: a patterns-of-care and outcome analysis. J Thorac Oncol 2013;8:1050–8.

19. Soldà F, Lodge M, Ashley S, et al. Stereotactic radiotherapy (SABR) for the treatment of primary non-small cell lung cancer; systematic review and comparison with a surgical cohort. Radiother Oncol 2013;109(1):1–7.

20. Kandioler D, Kromer E, Tuchler H, et al. Long-term results after repeated surgical removal of pulmonary metastases. Ann Thorac Surg 1998;65:909–12.

21. Gazelle GS, Goldberg SN, Solbiati L, et al. Tumor ablation with radio-frequency energy. Radiology 2000;217:633–46.

22. National Cancer Institute: Cancer Therapy Evaluation Program. Common terminology criteria for adverse events. Version 4.0. Available at: http://ctep.cancer. gov/protocolDevelopment/electronic_applications/ctc. htm. Accessed August 2, 2012.

23. Hiraki T, Gobara H, Mimura H, et al. Does tumor type affect local control by radiofrequency ablation in the lungs? Eur J Radiol 2010;74:136–41.

24. Lencioni R, Crocetti L, Cioni R, et al. Radiofrequency ablation of pulmonary tumors response evaluation: a prospective, intension-to-treat, multicenter clinical trial (the "RAPTURE" study). Lancet Oncol 2008;9: 621–8.

25. Singnurkar A, Solomon SB, Gonen M, et al. 18F-FDG PET/CT for the prediction and detection of local recurrence after radiofrequency ablation of malignant lung lesions. J Nucl Med 2010;51:1833–40.

26. Yamakado K, Hase S, Matsuoka T, et al. Radiofrequency ablation for the treatment of unresectable lung metastases in patients with colorectal cancer: a multicenter study in Japan. J Vasc Interv Radiol 2007;18:393–8.

27. Yan TD, King J, Sjarif A, et al. Percutaneous radiofrequency ablation of pulmonary metastases from

colorectal carcinoma: prognostic determinants for survival. Ann Surg Oncol 2006;13:1529–37.

28. Okuma T, Matsuoka T, Okamura T, et al. 18F-FDG small animal PET for monitoring the therapeutic effect of CT-guided radiofrequency ablation on implanted VX2 lung tumors in rabbits. J Nucl Med 2006;47:1351–8.

29. Yi CA, Lee KS, Kim BT, et al. Tissue characterization of solitary pulmonary nodule: comparative study between helical dynamic CT and integrated PET/CT. J Nucl Med 2006;47:443–50.

30. Rohren EM, Turkington TG, Coleman RE. Clinical application of OET in oncology. Radiology 2004; 231:305–32.

31. Keider Z, Haim N, Guralnik L, et al. PET/CT using 18F-FDG in suspected lung cancer recurrence: diagnostic value and impact on patient management. J Nucl Med 2004;45:1640–6.

32. Gupta NC, Graeber GM, Rogers JS, et al. Comparative efficacy of positron emission tomography with FDG and computed tomographic scanning in preoperative staging of non-small cell lung cancer. Ann Surg 1999;220:286–91.

33. Marom EM, Sarvis S, Herndon JE, et al. T1 lung cancers: sensitivity of diagnosis with fluorodeoxyglucose PET. Radiology 2001;223:453–9.

34. Vansteenkiste JF, Stroobants SG. The role of positron emission tomography with 18F-fluoro-2-deoxy-D-glucose in respiratory oncology. Eur Respir J 2001;17:802–20.

35. Gould MK, Maclean CC, Kuschner WG, et al. Accuracy of positron emission tomography for diagnosis of pulmonary nodules and mass lesions: a meta-analysis. JAMA 2001;285:914–24.

36. Fischer BM, Mortensen J, Hojgaard L. Positron emission tomography in the diagnosis and staging of lung cancer: a systematic, quantitative review. Lancet Oncol 2001;2:659–66.

37. Higuchi M, Hasegawa T, Osugi J, et al. Prognostic impact of FDG-PET in surgically treated pathological stage I lung adenocarcinoma. Ann Thorac Cardiovasc Surg 2014;20:185–91.

38. Shiono S, Abiko M, Okazaki T, et al. Positron emission tomography for predicting recurrence in stage I lung adenocarcinoma: standardized uptake value corrected by mean liver standardized uptake value. Eur J Cardiothorac Surg 2011;40:1165–9.

39. Ambrogi MC, Lucchi M, Dini P, et al. Percutaneous radiofrequency ablation of lung tumours: results in the mid-term. Eur J Cardiothorac Surg 2006;30: 177–83.

40. Padhani AR, Ollivier L. The RECIST (Response Evaluation Criteria in Solis Tumors) criteria: implications for diagnostic radiologists. Br J Radiol 2001;74: 983–6.

41. Abe Y, Matsuzawa T, Fujiwara T, et al. Clinical assessment of therapeutic effects on cancer using 18F-2-fluoro-2-deoxy-D-glucose and positron emission tomography: preliminary study of lung cancer. Int J Radiat Oncol Biol Phys 1990;19:1005–10.

42. Akhurst T, Downey RJ, Ginsberg MS, et al. An initial experience with FDG-PET in the imaging of residual disease after induction therapy for lung cancer. Ann Thorac Surg 2001;73:259–64.

43. Frank A, Lefkowitz D, Jaeger S, et al. Decision logic for retreatment of asymptomatic lung cancer recurrence based on positron emission tomography findings. Int J Radiat Oncol Biol Phys 1995; 32:1495–512.

44. Herbert ME, Lowe VJ, Hoffman JM, et al. Positron emission tomography in the pretreatment evaluation and follow-up of non-small cell lung cancer patients treated with radiotherapy: preliminary findings. Am J Clin Oncol 1996;19:416–21.

45. Patz EF Jr, Connolly J, Hendon J. Prognostic value of thoracic FDG PET imaging after treatment for non-small cell lung cancer. AJR Am J Roentgenol 2000;174:769–77.

46. Okuma T, Okamura T, Matsuoka T, et al. Fluorine-18-fluorodeoxyglucose positron emission tomography for assessment of patients with unresectable recurrent or metastatic lung cancers after CT-guided radiofrequency ablation: preliminary results. Ann Nucl Med 2006;20:115–20.

47. De Baere T, Risse O, KUoch V, et al. Adverse events during radiofrequency treatment of 582 hepatic tumors. AJR Am J Roentgenol 2003;181:695–700.

Fluorodeoxyglucose-PET/ Computed Tomography– Guided Biopsy

Juliano J. Cerci, PhD[a],*, Elena Tabacchi, MD[b],
Mateos Bogoni, MD[a]

KEYWORDS

• FDG-PET/CT • PET/CT • Guided biopsy • Cancer • Oncology

KEY POINTS

• PET/CT results often guide or lead to changes in therapy. The positive findings should whenever possible be confirmed by histology.
• PET/CT-guided biopsy offers a feasible new approach of potential value in optimizing the diagnostic yield of biopsies.
• PET/CT-guided biopsy is especially indicated in patients with only metabolic lesion but no anatomic correspondent lesion.
• PET/CT-guided biopsy might be performed in oncologic patients with metastatic disease in whom tumor transformation/mutation is suspected.
• PET/CT-guided biopsy might be performed in patients with new multiple lesions in a patient not known to have malignancy or who has had a prolonged remission or more than one primary malignancy.

HISTORY OF IMAGE-GUIDED BIOPSY

For the characterization of a suspected neoplastic lesion a sample of tissue needs to be collected for histologic analysis. The procedure of obtaining a tissue sample is usually carried out with the aid of an excisional biopsy (the whole lesion is removed) or with an incisional biopsy (only a part of the lesion is sampled) with or without an imaging method guiding the procedure. The first description of percutaneous biopsy using needles was given by Kun[1] in 1847, and only a few decades later, Hopper[2] described the first reports of imaging methods (ie, fluoroscopy) as guidance for biopsies. In the 1970s the use of thinner needles allowed much safer biopsies[3] and the accuracy of diagnosis and staging of cancer was improved by the guidance of ultrasound (US) and computed tomography (CT) in biopsy.[4] The imaging method of choice for guiding the biopsy depends mainly on the type of lesion and location of the lesion that needs to be sampled.[4]

Ultrasound-Guided Biopsy

US is widely applied in percutaneous needle biopsy, particularly in superficial tissue[5] and abdominal lesions. Advantages of this method are no radiation exposure to the patient, large availability, and low costs. Limitations are poor visualization of deep structures, the possible presence of air or bones hampering correct visualization of the lesion, and soft tissue attenuation in overweight patients.[2]

Computed Tomography–Guided Biopsy

In the 1960s Godfrey Hounsfield started assembling the first CT[6] and in 1971 performed the first

The authors have nothing to disclose.
[a] Quanta Diagnóstico e Terapia, Diagnostic and Therapy Clinic, Rua Almirante Tamandaré 1000, 4100400, Alto da XV - Curitiba, Paraná, Brazil; [b] Nuclear Medicine Unit, S. Orsola-Malpighi Hospital, Pavillion 30, via Massarenti 9, 40138, Bologna, Italy
* Corresponding author.
E-mail address: cercijuliano@hotmail.com

PET Clin 11 (2016) 57–64
http://dx.doi.org/10.1016/j.cpet.2015.08.001
1556-8598/16/$ – see front matter © 2016 Elsevier Inc. All rights reserved.

CT scan on a patient. By 1975, different CT scanner models were already available, performing full-body scans once the new fan-beam scanners with multiple detectors were developed. This new generation of CT scanners resulted in a decrease of the scanning time (around 5 seconds) and better image quality,[6] which allowed radiologists to sample tissues at sites previously considered inaccessible. In the late 1980s the single-slice helical CT scanner was introduced. It allowed faster scanning and better image quality, but it was not ideal for preventing movement artifacts or for covering large longitudinal areas. This problem was solved in the late 1990s with the multislice helical CT scanners, where several overlapping helixes supplied the computer for imaging reconstruction and provided thinner slices in comparison with the old slice scanner.[7] Advantages of this method for guiding biopsies are great anatomic spatial resolution, great characterization of solid including lung lesions, large availability, and low costs. Nevertheless, patient exposure to radiation still poses as an inherent limitation to the method.

MRI-Guided Biopsy

The first report of MRI-guided biopsy of head and neck lesions was published in 1986 by Mueller and colleagues.[8] This technique is preferable in abdominal, soft tissue, and bone biopsies, especially for lesions poorly visualized by CT or US.[9] MRI can be performed instead of CT when radiation exposure is a concern, in case of allergy to iodinated contrast agents, but the presence of the magnetic field of MRI requires special instrumentation. Specific indications of MRI-guided biopsy are subdiaphragmatic lesions and musculoskeletal lesions.[10]

MRI guidance is generally not indicated for chest lesions because of the poor visualization of pneumothorax, which is the main complication of thoracic puncturing.[10]

PET/Computed Tomography–Guided Biopsy

PET/CT combines the anatomic information from CT with PET metabolic characterization.[11] The clinical application of 18F-fluorodeoxyglucose (FDG) PET started in 1990s. 18F FDG-PET is helpful to differentiate malignant lesions that have usually high uptake from associated inflammation and atelectasis that have lower or no FDG uptake. However, active inflammation or infectious disease might also present FDG uptake.

Musculoskeletal lesions and large malignant lesions can be heterogeneous with areas of viable cells and necrosis. In that sense 18F FDG-PET/CT is able to guide biopsy to the area of highest 18F FDG uptake and major probability of viable neoplastic cells.[11,12]

The first studies on 18F FDG-PET/CT–guided biopsy were published in 2008 by O'Sullivan and colleagues[13] in musculoskeletal lesions. Klaeser and colleagues[14] published the result of their initial experiences with 12 patients, obtaining representative samples in 92% of the cases without major complications. The same conclusions were obtained by the study of Govindarajan and colleagues.[15] Tatli and colleagues[16] obtained good diagnostic results using PET/CT-guided biopsy of abdominal lesions and Klaeser and coworkers[14] reported a 56% clinical impact rate from PET/CT-guided biopsy in 20 patients with active bone lesions.

In 2012 our group used 18F FDG-PET/CT guidance for the biopsy of 130 lesions in different anatomic sites, and obtained representative tissue samples in 98.5% of the total number of lesions. Of the 130 lesions, 18% (23 of 180) were referred to PET/CT after a nondiagnostic CT-guided biopsy. Malignancy was diagnosed after PET/CT-guided biopsy in 21 of 23 lesions.[13] Similar results were obtained by Purandare and colleagues[17] in a study conduced in 122 patients.

Other studies[11,12] confirm the great value of PET/CT as the imaging method of choice for guiding biopsy procedures. Novel PET radiopharmaceuticals are also being investigated for guiding biopsies.[12,17]

TECHNICAL PROCEDURE OF FLUORODEOXYGLUCOSE-PET/COMPUTED TOMOGRAPHY–GUIDED BIOPSY

PET/CT-guided biopsy is an efficient diagnostic tool[17–21] that involves the previous administration of FDG and the subsequent PET/CT scan (60–90 minutes later). It is recommended but not necessary to perform the biopsy procedure in the same institution or scanner where the PET/CT images were acquired. However, if performed in different timing and scans the patient's position during the biopsy should be the same position in which PET/CT images were obtained, and images should be aligned manually to match intraprocedural CT images.[22]

Indications

Percutaneous biopsy might be considered but is not limited to patients with the following findings on imaging:

- New, enlarging, or PET-positive solitary pulmonary lesion (>1.0 cm) that is not amenable to diagnosis by bronchoscopy, or CT shows it is unlikely to be accessible by bronchoscopy.

- New, enlarging, or PET-positive lesion (>1.0 cm) that is suspicious for malignancy (lung, hepatic, breast, pancreas, spleen, adrenal, kidney, soft tissue, bone, and lymph node).
- New multiple lesions in patients with not known malignancy or with prolonged remission or more than one primary malignancy.
- Patients with lymphoma, breast, or lung cancer with metastatic disease where tumor transformation or mutation is suspected.

Contraindications

The most common contraindication is a lack of a safe path to perform biopsy. Prothrombin time, activated partial thromboplastin time, and platelet count should be checked preoperatively and oral anticoagulants should be stopped before biopsy in accordance with the published guidelines on perioperative anticoagulation. Relative contraindications include platelet count less than 100,000 per milliliter, and activated partial thromboplastin time ratio or prothrombin time ratio greater than 1.4. High-risk patients should not have a biopsy performed as an outpatient procedure.

Type of Biopsies

Biopsies may be classified according to type of access (percutaneous, bronchoscopic, laparoscopic, open surgery biopsies), and the tissue type of the sample obtained (cytologic or histologic). Percutaneous biopsies consist of fine-needle aspiration (FNA) biopsy and cutting or core biopsy.[23,24] FNA needles are usually 20 to 25 gauge and provide cells suitable for cytologic and microbiologic examination. Core biopsy needles are usually larger disposable needles (18–20 gauge) with outer cannula (metal tube) and inner, notched rod in which a tissue specimen is cut, trapped, and withdrawn (**Fig. 1**) and provides cores of tissue suitable for histologic examination. Automated core needles are available and provide a more efficient and easier way to get the specimens (**Fig. 2**).

FNA and core biopsies can be performed using a single needle technique (a single needle is directly advanced into the lesion and multiple passes provide multiple samples) or using a coaxial technique that includes initial placement of a guiding needle at the edge of the target lesion, followed by the introduction of a biopsy needle through guiding needle to sample the lesion without need of multiple passes to place the needle in the target lesion (**Fig. 3**). The anticipated

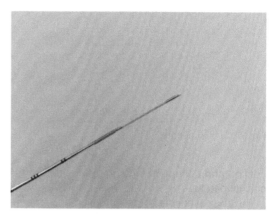

Fig. 1. Cutting or core biopsy needle in which a tissue specimen is cut, trapped, and withdrawn.

needle path is calculated on the CT console by extrapolating the path of the needle to the lesion.[18]

Procedure Description

Standard PET/CT images are acquired according to protocols described in national and international guidelines. FDG-PET/CT images are interpreted by imaging physicians with expertise in PET/CT imaging. After acquisition of the FDG-PET/CT images, the biopsy site and needle path are identified according to the location of the lesion and its relationship to anatomic structures.

Patients are positioned and immobilized according to the location of the lesion and the approach for the biopsy procedure. After completion of asepsis and antisepsis, local anesthesia is performed. Conscious sedation might be required when patients are anxious or noncooperative. The need for general anesthesia is uncommon.

If the coaxial technique is chosen, a suitable coaxial needle is inserted at the site previously identified. The angle and direction of the needle are adjusted according to the position of the suspicious lesion under the guidance of CT fluoroscopic imaging or CT acquisition. After placing the tip of the coaxial needle at the edge of the lesion, PET/CT images are acquired in one bed position to

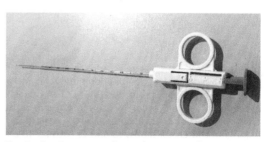

Fig. 2. Semiautomated core biopsy needle.

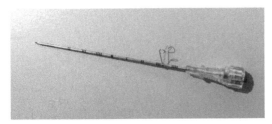

Fig. 3. Coaxial needle.

confirm and document the correct position of the coaxial needle.

The coaxial needle core is removed and a semi-automatic biopsy needle is inserted. The location of the needle is confirmed under fluoroscopy/CT scan and the biopsy site is imaged for documentation. If the lesion is small or difficult to be differentiated from important structures, such as peripheral vessels, contrast-enhanced CT can be used for optimization of the images. Then, the specimens are cut and drawn at 1- or 2-cm fragments. Three or four specimens are collected. After needle removal, manual compression at the puncture site should be applied during 2 to 5 minutes. The specimens are fixed in 10% formalin and sent for histopathologic examination. Intraoperative histopathologic examination with frozen sections is useful to reduce the need of performing repeat biopsies caused by sampling error.

Patients are observed for at least 3 hours after the procedure to ensure hemodynamic stability and monitoring the respiratory condition. CT is performed immediately and 3 hours after the biopsy procedure in patients in whom the needle punctured the pleura, liver, or stomach wall during the biopsy procedure.

Types of Access

Direct access

This is the simplest way to obtain a specimen and it is usually performed whenever possible. Caution should be taken when, for example, a lesion is suspicious for sarcoma; the needle should be placed along the planned surgical access for resecting the lesion because of the possibility of tumor cell seeding along the needle tract.[25–27] Direct access is illustrated in (**Fig. 4**).

To approach to lung lesion, generally the shortest intercostal route is taken during lung biopsies, avoiding pulmonary fissures, bullous lesions, and

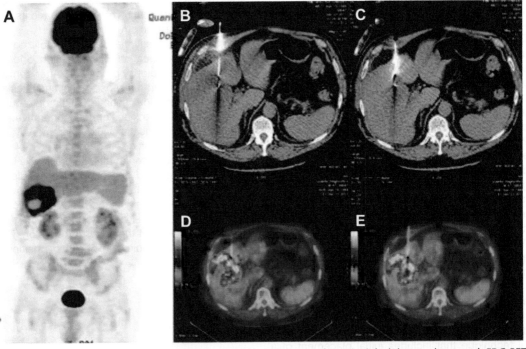

Fig. 4. A 52-year-old man with abdominal pain and a large lesion on hepatic right lobe on ultrasound. FDG-PET/CT maximum intensity projection (MIP) (*A*) and axial PET/CT images (*D* and *E*) revealed heterogeneous FDG uptake in the right lobe liver lesion measuring 121 mm in the largest diameter. The patient was positioned in the prone position. Direct abdominal access was the easiest path to the area of highest uptake in the medial border of the lesion and chosen for biopsy (*B* and *C*) with an 18-gauge needle. Histology and immunohistochemistry revealed adenocarcinoma.

emphysematous areas.[28,29] It is preferable to access the lesion through a nonaerated route to avoid the risk of pneumothorax. When the lesion is cavitary or has air bronchogram, the biopsy is obtained from the wall of the lesion or the most solid part of the lesion.[29]

Oblique access

If a major vessel or a bone is along the way of a planned trajectory for the biopsy, various maneuvers can be helpful, such as changing the position of the patient's leg or arm, taking a more medial or lateral path (**Fig. 5**), rotating the patient, puncturing the patient from the opposite side if feasible, and changing the respiration. A lesion that cannot be accessed can also be approached using angled insertion of the biopsy needle in the craniocaudal axis. Coronal and sagittal multiplanar CT reconstructions are useful to determine the required angulation and the skin entry site.

Bone and transbone approach

Bone biopsy and transbone approach involves needle placement through the bone using the coaxial needle technique (**Fig. 6**). The administration of a local anesthetic on the periosteum minimizes the discomfort associated with the procedure. In the transsternal approach, intravenous administration of a contrast may be needed during the procedure to help identify the vascular structures.

Transpulmonary approach to the mediastinal lesions

This approach is used when a mediastinal lesion cannot be approached by the extrapleural route.[30–32] The patient is positioned according to the location of the lesion and the coaxial needle passes through the lung parenchyma and two layers of visceral pleura. Other precautions are similar to a lung biopsy.

ACUTE COMPLICATIONS OF BIOPSY PROCEDURES

Physicians should be able to identify and appropriately manage the complications of biopsy procedures. Resuscitation facilities and chest drain

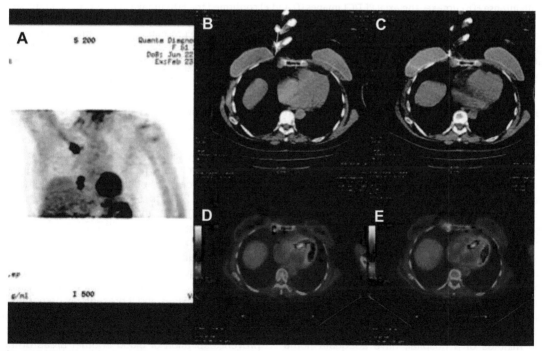

Fig. 5. A 61-year-old man with a history of breast cancer submitted to surgery, chemotherapy, and radiotherapy. Patient presented weight loss and a palpable infraclavicular lymph node. FDG-PET/CT MIP image (*A*) and axial PET/CT images (*D* and *E*) revealed infraclavicular and right internal mammary lymph nodes with intense FDG uptake. The patient was positioned in the prone position with thorax immobilized. Direct access to the lesion with higher uptake was the easiest and safest path to the lesion and chosen for biopsy (*B* and *C*). A single bed position of FDG-PET/CT (*D* and *E*) was acquired to confirm needle position in an area within FDG uptake. Biopsy was performed with direct access of lesion with highest FDG uptake in internal mammary lymph node with 18-gauge needle (*B* and *C*). Histology and immunohistochemistry revealed breast cancer recurrence. Material was further analyzed to evaluation of tumor mutation.

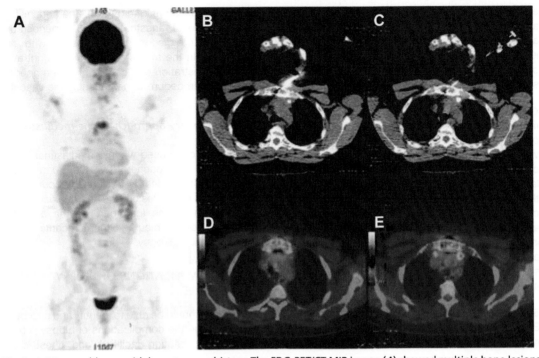

Fig. 6. A 68-year-old man with breast cancer history. The FDG-PET/CT MIP image (*A*) showed multiple bone lesions with intense FDG uptake. The axial PET/CT images (*D* and *E*) confirmed the FDG uptake in a lytic lesion in the sternum, the lesion with higher uptake. In a patient with multiple lesions, choosing a representative lesion for biopsy takes into account the FDG uptake and the risk of complications from the procedure. Because the sternum lesion presents the bigger lesion and also the higher uptake area, a bone biopsy technique was used to perform the sternum biopsy with an 18-gauge needle (*B* and *C*). Histology and immunohistochemistry revealed breast cancer recurrence.

equipment should be immediately available. When a complication occurs, heart rate, blood pressure, and oxygen saturation should be monitored and recorded. Percutaneous biopsies can be performed safely on an outpatient basis. However, high-risk patients should not have a biopsy performed as outpatient. A postbiopsy image (supine chest radiograph, CT of the region of concern) should be performed at least 1 hour after the procedure to assess the presence of pneumothorax or other complications. During the informed consent process, patients should be made aware of potential delayed complications and given verbal and written instructions to return if they become symptomatic. When biopsies are performed on an outpatient basis, patients should live within 30 minutes of a hospital, have adequate home support, and have access to a telephone.

A postbiopsy image (supine chest radiograph, CT of the region of concern) should be performed at least 1 hour after the procedure to assess the presence of complications: pneumothorax, hemorrhage, hemothorax, and hematoma are the most common,[2,33–35] whereas hemomediastinum, cardiac tamponade, air embolism, vasovagal reaction, emphysema, and tumor seeding are less common.[33,35]

Physicians should audit their own practice at least annually and calculate their complication rates to inform patients before consent is given. The incidence of postbiopsy pneumothorax ranges from 27% to 54% in most of the large series (**Fig. 7**) and although most of these cases can be managed conservatively, about 3% to 15% of patients require chest tube placement.[32,36,37] In our experience less than 1% of the cases require intervention.[18]

Pulmonary hemorrhage occurs in 5.0% to 16.9% of the cases and it presents as hemoptysis in only 1.2% to 5.0%.[23] Patients should be placed in the decubitus position with biopsy side down to prevent aspiration of blood in other areas of the lung.[35,38]

The risk of pulmonary hemorrhage increases in patients with chronic inflammatory cavities caused by the presence of hypertrophied bronchial arteries, with vascular tumors, with centrally located lesions, with pulmonary hypertension, and with abnormal coagulation profile.[23] In vascular lesions and in patients with bleeding

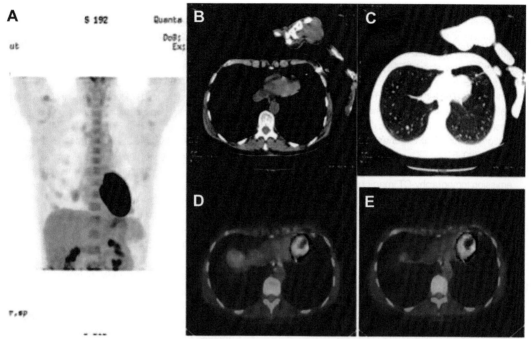

Fig. 7. Lung biopsy presenting small pneumothorax. This 67-year-old man with previously treated colon cancer presented with pulmonary nodules on follow-up CT imaging 2 years later. The FDG-PET/CT MIP (*A*) and axial view (*D*, *E*) showed moderate uptake in the left lower lobe lung lesion measuring 12 mm in largest dimension on CT. The patient was positioned in the prone position with the arms immobilized in a comfortable position (*B* and *C*). A small pneumothorax occurred following the biopsy (*C*). During follow-up, the 3-hour imaging control revealed a stable pneumothorax in an asymptomatic patient. Patient was discharged and remained asymptomatic during follow-up. Histology revealed tuberculosis.

disorders, small-caliber needles should be used to reduce the risk of severe hemorrhage.[23]

Significant hematoma and hemothorax are rare, but may develop if the intercostal or internal mammary arteries are injured during the biopsy procedure. Pneumorrhachis, the presence of intraspinal air, has been rarely reported after anesthetic interventions.[38]

Air embolism is a very rare complication[39] caused by the introduction of ambient air into the pulmonary vein with the biopsy needle, or by the formation of a bronchovenous fistula along the needle path or in the biopsy cavity. Factors associated with air embolisms are coughing during the procedure, biopsy of consolidated lung, cavitary or cystic lesions, associated vasculitis, and use of the coaxial technique.[37] To prevent air embolism, the guiding needle should never be left without the inner stylet. During exchange of inner stylet with the biopsy needle, the hub of the guiding needle should be covered with the finger or thumb.[37]

REFERENCES

1. Kun M. A new instrument for the diagnosis of tumors. Month J Med Sci 1847;7:853–4.

2. Hopper KD. Percutaneous, radiographically guided biopsy: a history. Radiology 1995;196:329–33.

3. Zornoza J, Snow J, Lukeman JM, et al. Aspiration biopsy of discrete pulmonary lesions using a new thin needle. Radiology 1977;123:519–20.

4. Interventional Radiology Grand Rounds. Society of Interventional Radiology, 2004. Available at: www.SIRweb.org. Accessed September 19, 2015.

5. Soudack M, Nachtigal A, Vladovski E, et al. Sonographically guided percutaneous needle biopsy of soft tissue masses with histopathologic correlation. J Ultrasound Med 2006;25(10):1271–7.

6. Robb WL. Perspective on the first 10 years of the CT scanner industry. Acad Radiol 2003;10(7):756–60.

7. Wesolowski JR, Lev MH. CT: history, technology, and clinical aspects. Semin Ultrasound CT MR 2005;26(6):376–9.

8. Mueller PR, Stark DD, Simeone JF, et al. MR-guided aspiration biopsy: needle design and clinical trials. Radiology 1986;161:605–9.

9. Kerimaa P, Marttila A, Hyvönen P, et al. MRI-guided biopsy and fine needle aspiration biopsy (FNAB) in the diagnosis of musculoskeletal lesions. Eur J Radiol 2013;82(12):2328–33.

10. Adam G, Bücker A, Nolte-Ernsting C, et al. Interventional MR imaging: percutaneous abdominal and

skeletal biopsies and drainages of the abdomen. Eur Radiol 1999;9(8):1471–8.

11. Kobayashi K, Bhargava P, Raja S, et al. Image-guided biopsy: what the interventional radiologist needs to know about PET/CT. Radiographics 2012; 32(5):1483–501.

12. Klaeser B, Mueller MD, Schmid RA, et al. PET-CT-guided interventions in the management of FDG-positive lesions in patients suffering from solid malignancies: initial experiences. Eur Radiol 2009; 19(7):1780–5.

13. O'Sullivan PJ, Rohren EM, Madewell JE. Positron emission tomography-CT imaging in guiding musculoskeletal biopsy. Radiol Clin North Am 2008;46(3): 475–86.

14. Klaeser B, Wiskirchen J, Wartenberg J, et al. PET/CT-guided biopsies of metabolically active bone lesions: applications and clinical impact. Eur J Nucl Med Mol Imaging 2010;37(11):2027–36.

15. Govindarajan MJ, Nagaraj KR, Kallur KG, et al. PET/CT guidance for percutaneous fine needle aspiration cytology/biopsy. Indian J Radiol Imaging 2009; 19:208–9.

16. Tatli S, Gerbaudo VH, Mamede M, et al. Abdominal masses sampled at PET/CT-guided percutaneous biopsy: initial experience with registration of prior PET/CT images. Radiology 2010;256(1):305–11.

17. Purandare NC, Kulkarni AV, Kulkarni SS, et al. 18F-FDG PET/CT-directed biopsy: does it offer incremental benefit? Nucl Med Commun 2013;34(3):203–10.

18. Cerci JJ, Pereira Neto CC, Krauzer C, et al. The impact of coaxial core biopsy guided by FDG PET/CT in oncological patients. Eur J Nucl Med Mol Imaging 2013;40(1):98–103.

19. Slomka PJ. Software approach to merging molecular with anatomic information. J Nucl Med 2004; 45(Suppl 1):36S–45S.

20. Maintz JB, Viergever MA. A survey of medical image registration. Med Image Anal 1998;2(1):1–36.

21. Shekhar R, Walimbe V, Raja S, et al. Automated 3-dimensional elastic registration of whole-body PET and CT from separate or combined scanners. J Nucl Med 2005;46(9):1488–96.

22. Lindblom K. Diagnostic kidney puncture in cysts and tumors. Am J Roentgenol Radium Ther Nucl Med 1952;68:209–15.

23. Manhire A, Charig M, Clelland C, et al. Guidelines for radiologically guided lung biopsy. Thorax 2003; 58:920–36.

24. Cham MD, Lane ME, Henschke CI, et al. Lung biopsy: special techniques. Semin Respir Crit Care Med 2008;29:335–49.

25. Robertson EG, Baxter G. Tumour seeding following percutaneous needle biopsy: the real story! Clin Radiol 2011;66(11):1007–14.

26. Loughran CF, Keeling CR. Seeding of tumour cells following breast biopsy: a literature review. Br J Radiol 2011;84(1006):869–74.

27. Silva MA, Hegab B, Hyde C, et al. Needle track seeding following biopsy of liver lesions in the diagnosis of hepatocellular cancer: a systematic review and meta-analysis. Gut 2008;57(11):1592–6.

28. Wallace AB, Suh RD. Percutaneous transthoracic needle biopsy: special considerations and techniques used in lung transplant recipients. Semin Intervent Radiol 2004;21:247–58.

29. Bandoh S, Fujita J, Fukunaga Y, et al. Cavitary lung cancer with an aspergilloma-like shadow. Lung Cancer 1999;26:195–8.

30. Gupta S, Seaberg K, Wallace MJ, et al. Imaging-guided percutaneous biopsy of mediastinal lesions: different approaches and anatomic considerations. Radiographics 2005;25:763–88.

31. Klein JS, Salomon G, Stewart EA. Transthoracic needle biopsy with a coaxially placed 20-gauge automated cutting needle: results in 122 patients. Radiology 1996;198:715–20.

32. Moore EH. Technical aspects of needle aspiration lung biopsy: a personal perspective. Radiology 1998;208:303–18.

33. Diamantis A, Magiorkinis E, Koutselini H. Fine-needle aspiration (FNA) biopsy: historical aspects. Folia Histochem Cytobiol 2009;47(2):191–7.

34. Collings CL, Westcott JL, Banson NL, et al. Pneumothorax and dependent versus nondependent patient position after needle biopsy of the lung. Radiology 1999;210:59–64.

35. Wu CC, Maher MM, Shepard JA. Complications of CT-guided percutaneous needle biopsy of the chest: prevention and management. AJR Am J Roentgenol 2011;196:W678–82.

36. Cox JE, Chiles C, McManus CM, et al. Transthoracic needle aspiration biopsy: variables that affect risk of pneumothorax. Radiology 1999;212:165–8.

37. Tsai IC, Tsai WL, Chen MC, et al. CT-guided core biopsy of lung lesions: a primer. AJR Am J Roentgenol 2009;193:1228–35.

38. Oertel MF, Korinth MC, Reinges MH, et al. Pathogenesis, diagnosis and management of pneumorrhachis. Eur Spine J 2006;15(Suppl 5):636–43.

39. Hare SS, Gupta A, Goncalves AT, et al. Systemic arterial air embolism after percutaneous lung biopsy. Clin Radiol 2011;66:589–96.

Dual-time-point Imaging and Delayed-time-point Fluorodeoxyglucose-PET/ Computed Tomography Imaging in Various Clinical Settings

Sina Houshmand, MD[a,1], Ali Salavati, MD, MPH[a,b,1],
Eivind Antonsen Segtnan, BSc[c], Peter Grupe, MD[c],
Poul Flemming Høilund-Carlsen, MD, DMSc[c],
Abass Alavi, MD[a,*]

KEYWORDS

- FDG-PET/CT • Dual-time-point imaging • Cancer • Glucose-6-phosphatase • Inflammation

KEY POINTS

- Dual-time-point imaging (DTPI) and delayed-time-point imaging have been introduced to overcome the nonspecificity of the fluorodeoxyglucose (FDG)-PET.
- In addition to the distribution time of the radiotracer and level of blood glucose, which affect FDG accumulation in the target tissues, the decrease in the background activity in delayed time points leads to enhanced lesion detection.
- DTPI has been shown to be useful in both malignant and nonmalignant diseases, such as in the prognostication of patients with lung cancer, diagnosis of primary breast cancer, and detection of atherosclerotic plaques.
- Considering the pros and cons of DTPI in assessment of various diseases, the best approach for increasing the accuracy seems to be using DTPI selectively in the clinical setting.

INTRODUCTION

Fluorodeoxyglucose (FDG)-PET/computed tomography (CT) imaging enables clinicians to assess cancer biology and perform staging, restaging, and treatment monitoring of cancers.[1] FDG is an analogue of glucose with a missing hydroxyl group at the 2' position, which is substituted with positron-emitting fluorine 18, and is taken by the glucose transporter 1 (GLUT1) into the cell. After phosphorylation of FDG by hexokinase, an enzyme in the glycolytic pathway to FDG-6-phosphate,

Disclosure: The authors have nothing to disclose.
[a] Department of Radiology, University of Pennsylvania, 3400 Spruce Street, Philadelphia, PA 19104, USA;
[b] Department of Radiology, University of Minnesota, 420 Delaware Street Southeast, Minneapolis, MN 55455, USA; [c] Department of Nuclear Medicine, Odense University Hospital, Sdr. Boulevard 29, Odense C 5000, Denmark
[1] S. Houshmand and A. Salavati have contributed equally to this article.
* Corresponding author. Hospital of the University of Pennsylvania, 3400 Spruce Street, Philadelphia, PA 19104.
E-mail address: abass.alavi@uphs.upenn.edu

PET Clin 11 (2016) 65–84
http://dx.doi.org/10.1016/j.cpet.2015.07.003
1556-8598/16/$ – see front matter © 2016 Elsevier Inc. All rights reserved.

accumulation of this radiotracer eventually allows characterization of tumor biology and detection of various types of lesions, both malignant and benign. However, the specificity of FDG for malignancy is limited.[2] To improve the specificity of FDG for differentiation of malignant and benign lesions, dual-time-point imaging (DTPI) and delayed-time-point imaging techniques have been introduced.[3–5] In DTPI and delayed-time-point imaging the acquisition of the PET studies is done at 1 standard time point and repeated after a certain amount of time, and has been suggested to increase the accuracy of FDG-PET imaging for distinction between benign and malignant lesions.[3–6]

The time interval between injection of FDG and image acquisition determines the intensity of the FDG uptake and its clearance from the blood. The tissues with high levels of glycolysis activity convert FDG to FDG-6-phosphate and retain it. FDG-6-phosphate might remain unchanged or be dephosphorylated back to FDG by the glucose-6-phosphatase enzyme. The glucose-6-phosphatase enzyme is thought to be the cause of different patterns of FDG uptake in malignant versus nonmalignant cells because of lower levels of glucose-6-phosphatase in some cancerous cells and also greater demand for glucose (and therefore, FDG) caused by the high metabolic rate in these cells.[7] These characteristics could explain the continuous accumulation of FDG-6-phosphate in malignant cells at delayed time points.[8,9] In contrast, inflammatory and infectious processes are thought to have different FDG uptake patterns owing to the higher levels of glucose-6-phosphatase. As discussed earlier, differentiation between benign and malignant lesions based only on FDG uptake at 1 time point may not always be accurate.[7,10–12] It has been shown that FDG uptake increases with time in malignant

tumors, whereas it might do so in the inflammatory and nonmalignant tissues.[13] In addition, malignant cells bear higher numbers of glucose transporters and high levels of hexokinase enzyme, which enhances the effect mentioned earlier.[6,14] Several studies have used DTPI in normal and abnormal states, including in lung,[5,15–19] breast (Table 1),[20–25] head and neck,[3,26] and pancreatic[27] cancers; atherosclerosis (Fig. 1)[28,29]; and many other settings (Fig. 2).[30] The impact of this imaging technique on diagnosis, prognosis,[31] and treatment planning[32] has been assessed for different malignant and benign diseases,[33] and the benefits and pitfalls of DTPI are shown in Table 2.

This article reviews the applications of DTPI and delayed-time-point imaging in various clinical settings.

DYNAMIC CHANGES OF FLUORODEOXYGLUCOSE UPTAKE OVER TIME

The factors affecting the accumulation of FDG in the target tissue include distribution time of the tracer and level of the plasma glucose.[34] In addition, the decrease in the background activity over time enhances the contrast between target lesion and the surrounding tissues.[2] Malignant lesions and inflammatory processes are considered to have overlap and no specific number has been assigned as cutoff between these two entities.[35] In order to have a better understanding of these variations, it would be beneficial to know the physiologic uptake and dynamics of FDG at different time points.[35,36]

Cheng and colleagues[36–38] examined 59 patients with FDG-PET scans at 1, 2, and 3 hours postinjection, quantified FDG uptake in the normal tissues, and analyzed the background activity

Table 1
This table shows the average SUV_{max} of the primary lesions of patients with breast cancer at two time points ($SUV_{max}1$ and $SUV_{max}2$) and the percent change between these two time points ($\%\Delta SUV_{max}$). There are three groups of patients: Those with no metastases (Group 1), patients with local metastases (Group 2) and patients with distant metastases (Group 3). SUV_{max} in the primary lesion was the lowest in the group 1. In addition, the degree of increase in tumor metabolism over time in groups 2 and 3 were substantially higher compared to group 1. This observation demonstrates the role of early and delayed imaging in assessing tumor biology.

	Primary Breast Lesions in Patients Without Axillary or Distant Metastasis (Highly Differentiated)	Primary Breast Lesions in Patients with Axillary Metastasis (Intermediate Differentiation)	Primary Breast Lesions in Patients with Distant Metastasis (Highly Undifferentiated)	P
$SUV_{max}1$	2.9 ± 2.7	4.8 ± 3.9	7.7 ± 6.2	.01
$SUV_{max}2$	3.4 ± 2.4	5.3 ± 4.5	8.9 ± 7.1	.01
$\%\Delta SUV_{max}$	4.5 ± 4.2	9.4 ± 12.8	15.7 ± 10.8	>.05

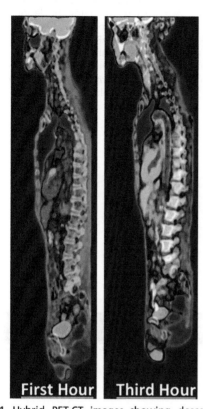

First Hour   Third Hour

Fig. 1. Hybrid PET-CT images showing descending aorta at first and third hours after injection of FDG. Decrease in the blood pool activity in the aorta can be noted over time. In contrast, aortic wall signal has increased and therefore contrast between the aorta and the blood pool has enhanced yielding higher visual scores at later time points.

clearance of these tissues. Blood pool, spleen, and liver (**Fig. 3**) were the 3 organs in which the FDG activity declined over time, whereas lymph nodes, pancreas, lung, and skeletal muscles decreased from first to second time points. Bone marrow and left ventricle FDG uptake increased over time. Some organs did not show any change over time, including parotid gland, thyroid, and prostate. These different patterns of change can be used for interpretation of studies done at short or long distribution time and also studies with different distribution times.

Basu and colleagues[39] investigated the changes of the FDG uptake over extended time periods (5 minutes, 1 hour, 2 hours, 4 hours, 6 hours, and 8 hours) in various normal and abnormal tissues of 3 patients with lung cancer and generated time-activity curves for each organ and lesion. The results showed declining pattern for normal tissues, including heart, liver, lung, large bowel, and small bowel, whereas neoplastic lesions, including primary tumor, metastatic sites,

and lymph nodes, increased over time. These findings show the importance of delayed-time-point imaging and also early and delayed tumor heterogeneity (**Fig. 4**). The variations in the slopes of the time-activity curves might reflect the tumor heterogeneity of examined lesions in patients with non–small cell lung cancer (NSCLC) (**Fig. 5**, see **Table 1**).

APPLICATIONS OF DUAL-TIME-POINT IMAGING IN MALIGNANT DISEASES
Lung

Diagnostic role of dual-time-point imaging in lung cancer
About 65% of the nodules found in the lungs are benign (mostly inflammatory reactions), and malignant lesions comprise only one-third of the pulmonary nodules.[40,41] FDG-PET/CT is a well-established imaging modality for diagnosis of lung cancer (**Figs. 6–9**) with some limitations reported in the literature, including false-positive and false-negative results.[4,5,42] However, over delayed times of 2 or 3 hours, the lymph nodes become clearer and easier to detect compared with 1-hour imaging.

Three systematic reviews and meta-analyses have calculated the diagnostic value of DTPI versus single-time-point imaging (STPI) in pulmonary nodules with similar results[15,43,44] of not having an additive value compared with STPI. Lin and colleagues[43] selected 11 studies with 788 patients and compared STPI versus DTPI. The area under the curve (AUC) for differentiation of malignant solitary pulmonary nodules from benign nodules was 0.839 for DTPI and 0.757 for STPI. They concluded that DTPI might be used for cases with equivocal results in STPI. Zhang and colleagues[44] in their meta-analysis included 415 patients from 8 studies. Compared with the gold standard, DTPI had a pooled sensitivity of 79% (95% confidence interval [CI], 74%–84%) and pooled specificity of 73% (95% CI, 65%–79%). STPI was 77% (95% CI, 71.9%–82.3%) sensitive and 59% (95% CI, 0.29–0.49) specific. Based on this meta-analysis, although similar in accuracy, DTPI seemed to be more specific. Barger and Nandalur[15] included 10 articles with 816 patients and the calculated pooled sensitivity for DTPI was 85% (95% CI, 82%–89%) and pooled specificity was 77% (95% CI, 72%–81%), which was similar to previously reported STPI ranges.[45] In conclusion, lack of additive value of DTPI compared with STPI was thought to be caused by the significant overlap in nodule size and heterogeneity between studies.

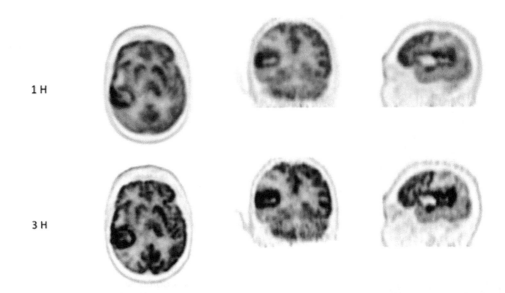

Diagnosis	Time point	MTV	SUVmax	SUV mean	Pvc SUVmean	TLG	Pvc TLG	Δ%pvc TLG
HGG	1 h	6.4	20.7	12.3	28	78.8	179.2	
	3 h	12.6	26.2	15.6	33.6	195.9	422.3	135

Fig. 2. Transaxial, coronal, and sagittal images of right temporal lobe high-grade glioma (HGG) acquired at 1 and 3 hours showing significant uptake at 1 hour at the tumor site, which increases substantially over time, as noted on the 3-hour image. The degree of increased activity over time in brain tumors reflects tumor aggressiveness and seems to correlate with patient outcome. Note the reduced cortical and subcortical metabolic activity ipsilateral to the tumor, which likely is caused by edema adjacent to these structures. This reduced activity is frequently noted in high-grade tumors and is not seen with lower grade malignancies. Also note the reduced activity in the left cerebellum, which is caused by the diaschisis effect noted with supratentorial diseases, including vascular accidents and brain tumors. By using segmentation techniques we generated the quantitative data in this patient (noted earlier). These parameters include metabolic tumor volume (MTV), maximal standardized uptake value (SUV_{max}), mean standardized uptake value (SUV_{mean}), partial volume corrected SUV_{mean} (pvcSUV_{mean}), total lesion glycolysis (TLG), and partial volume corrected TLG (pvcTLG). pvcTLG seemed to be superior to TLG, which might reflect the degree of aggressiveness of the brain tumor. We expect such an approach to prove to be superior to standard measurements that are based on correcting for partial volume effect of, as well as the size of, the lesion. Adapting this powerful methodology will allow the accurate determination of the degree of aggressiveness of this serious cancer, which is likely to affect the optimal management of patients with brain tumors.

Prognostic role of dual-time-point imaging in lung cancer

Some studies have assessed the predictive value of DTPI and delayed-time-point imaging in lung malignancies.[46–48] In one study,[47] changes in the maximal standardized uptake value (SUV_{max}) from the first hour to 90 minutes have been identified as a strong independent predictive factor. An increase in the SUV_{max} of more than 25% predicted shorter overall survival (OS). In contrast, Kim and colleagues,[49] in their study of surgically resected early stage NSCLC, noted that the change in the SUV_{max} may not be predictive, whereas SUV_{max} at the first time point was significantly predictive for OS and disease-free survival ($P<.05$).

A more recent study[46] assessed the prognostic value of DTPI in a group of patients with NSCLC by calculating the increase in the SUV_{max} from one time point to another and noted that an increase of standardized uptake value (SUV) of more than 1 unit was the best prognosticator for progression-free survival (PFS). In the group of patients with less than a 1-unit increase, the 3-year PFS and OS were 61.6% and 87.8%, respectively. The other group with greater than a

Table 2
Studies that implemented DTPI and delayed-time-point imaging

Study (First Author, Year)	Clinical Setting	Affected Organ	N	Parameters, Evaluated	Findings and Conclusions
Shinozaki et al,[93] 2014	Staging of preoperative lung cancer	Lung cancer	100	SUV_{max}, RI	Early phase FDG-PET changed the staging of tumors to an upper level in 10% and downstaged 5% of them
Cheng et al,[16] 2014	Diagnostic value of serial FDG uptake in malignant vs benign lung lesions	Lung cancer	43	SUV_{max}, RI	2-h and 3-h SUV_{max} similarly outperformed first-hour SUV_{max}. The optimum cutoff values for malignant benign differentiation were 3.24, 3.67, and 4.21 for first, second, and third hours. Third-hour SUV_{max} had the best overall performance with accuracy of 88.8%. Delayed imaging significantly enhanced the quality of image
Garcia Vicente et al,[21] 2014	Nodal staging and staging detection of extra-axillary involvement in breast cancer	Breast cancer	75	Visual, SUV_{max}	Sensitivity and specificity of visual assessment were 87.3% and 75%, respectively. Early and delayed SUV_{max} of 0.9 and 0.95 had the best sensitivity for first and second time points, respectively. 1.95 and 2.75 were the most specific values for SUV_{max} at first and second time points, respectively
Lee et al,[94] 2014	Differential diagnosis of thyroid incidentaloma	Thyroid incidentaloma	29	SUV_{max}, RI	SUV at second time point and RI were able to discriminate between benign and malignant thyroid lesions. SUV at the second time point with a cutoff of 3.9 was 87.5% sensitive and 75% specific. RI >12.5% was expected to be malignant
Kaneko et al,[17] 2013	Differentiation of benign pulmonary lesions (tuberculous and nontuberculous) and primary lung cancers	Lung cancer	81	SUV_{max}, RI	Benign pulmonary lesions and primary lung cancer lesions both had similar high RIs (mean ± SD 33.6 ± 22.6 and 32.5 ± 23.7, $P = .95$). Both tuberculous and nontuberculous lesions had high RI values. Benign lesions tended to show lower RIs in higher SUVs at first time point, whereas malignant lesions had persistent high RIs without relationship to SUV. No significant difference between malignant and benign lesions

(continued on next page)

Table 2
(continued)

Study (First Author, Year)	Clinical Setting	Affected Organ	N	Parameters, Evaluated	Findings and Conclusions
Li et al,[88] 2012	Regional nodal staging in NSCLC using DTPI for differentiation vs tubercular granulomatous tissues	Lung cancer	39	RI	Difference in the RI in the benign and malignant lesions was not statistically significant. FDG-PET combined with CT attenuation improved the diagnostic specificity and accuracy. DTPI had limited applicability for lymph node differentiation
Satoh et al,[48] 2012	DTPI for evaluation of prognosis and risk factors for recurrence in stage I stereotactic body radiation therapy–treated NSCLC	Lung cancer	57	SUV_{max}, RI	Three-year overall survival was 63.4%. SUV_{max} did not change any prognostic measure. RI predicted higher numbers of distant metastasis and fewer local recurrences and regional lymph node metastases
Kim et al,[52] 2012	DTPI for lymph node staging in NSCLC	Lung cancer	69	SUV_{max}, RI	Delayed SUV_{max} was more accurate than RI and early SUV_{max} in the lymph node–based analysis. DTPI could increase the diagnostic accuracy for lymph node staging of NSCLC
Kim et al,[49] 2011	Prognosis of early stage NSCLC using DTPI	Lung cancer	66	SUV_{max}, $\%\Delta SUV_{max}$	Overall survival and disease-free survival in patients with $SUV_{max} \leq 5.75$ was better than in the group with $SUV_{max} > 5.75$. $\%\Delta SUV_{max}$ did not have prognostic value. SUV_{max} (early and delayed) predicted overall survival. $\%\Delta SUV_{max}$ had limited prognostic value
Kim et al,[95] 2011	Evaluation of predictive value of DTPI in N1 status in NSCLC	Lung cancer	70	SUV_{max}, $\%\Delta SUV_{max}$	DTPI was not able to predict pathologic N1 status in NSCLC
MacDonald et al,[96] 2011	Evaluation of solitary pulmonary nodules with initial standard uptake <2.5	Lung cancer	54	SUV_{max}, RI	DTPI with RI analysis is useful for evaluation of solitary pulmonary nodules with $SUV_{max} < 2.5$. Prolongation of delay time from 120 to 180 min did not add any value

Study	Purpose	Cancer type	No.	Parameters	Findings
Lee et al,[97] 2011	Detection of liver metastasis in patients with colorectal cancer using DTPI	Colorectal cancer	39	Visual, SUV, TLR, percentage changes of SUV and TLR	SUV and TLR of metastatic lesions were higher in the delayed images. Visual analysis detected 77% of lesions on early and 87% of lesions on delayed images. DTPI is promising for detection of liver metastasis in colorectal cancer
Yoon et al,[98] 2013	Neoadjuvant chemoradiation response of locally advanced rectal cancer	Colorectal cancer	61	SUV_{max}, RI, dual-point index	RI and dual-point index remained as significant predictors in the multivariate analysis. Delay index was 86.7% sensitive, 87% specific, with PPV of 68.4% and NPV of 95.2% and accuracy of 86.9%. Dual-point post-chemoradiation therapy PET/CT study is a better predictor of pathologic tumor than single-time-point pre-chemoradiation therapy and post-chemoradiation therapy PET/CT
Toriihara et al,[99] 2013	Salivary gland tumor characterization	Salivary gland tumor	40	SUV_{max}, RI	No significant difference was noted between early and delayed SUV_{max}. Dual-time-point FDG-PET is not useful for this purpose
Nakayama et al,[100] 2013	Differentiating lymph nodes between malignant lymphoma and benign lesions	Lymphoma	84	SUV_{max} difference between early and delayed SUV_{max}, RI	Delayed parameters were significantly higher in malignant lymphoma than in benign lesions. Delayed FDG uptake parameters were useful indices for differentiation of malignant lymphoma from benign lesions
Matthiessen et al,[58] 2013	Evaluating DTPI in large locoregional recurrences following electrochemotherapy for breast cancer	Breast cancer	11	SUV_{max}	1-h and 3-h delayed imaging is a promising technique for assessment of electrochemotherapy-treated breast cancer recurrences on the skin
Costantini et al,[101] 2013	Assessment of DTPI in pediatric malignancies	Pediatric malignancies	21	SUV_{max}, RI	Average SUV increased from 7.3 to 10.9 in malignant cases, whereas it changed from 4.5 to 4.2 in benign lesions. Average RI for malignant lesions was 37.1% vs −9.9% for benign cases. Cutoff value of 10% for RI showed sensitivity and specificity of 77% and 80% respectively

(continued on next page)

Table 2
(continued)

Study (First Author, Year)	Clinical Setting	Affected Organ	N	Parameters, Evaluated	Findings and Conclusions
Choi et al,[60] 2013	Differentiating extrahepatic cholangiocarcinoma from benign disease using DTPI	Cholangiocarcinoma	39	SUV_{max}, %ΔSUV_{max}, ratio of SUV_{max} and %ΔSUV_{max} in comparison with average SUV of right hepatic lobe	Significant difference in SUV_{max}1 in benign and malignant lesions (5.43 ± 4.66 vs 2.26 ± 0.83, P = .003). Same results for SUV_{max}2 (6.02 ± 5.26 vs 2.26 ± 0.76, P = .002). No significant difference in other parameters was noted. No added benefit of DTPI was seen
Shum et al,[102] 2012	DTPI for assessment of esophageal squamous cell carcinoma	Esophageal cancer	26	SUV_{max}, RI	Combination of early SUV_{max} ≥ 2.5 or RI ≥ 10% had a sensitivity of 96.2%, which was the highest. Higher specificity was noted when combination of SUV_{max} ≥ 2.5 and RI ≥ 10% or SUV_{max} ≥ 2.5 alone was implemented. DTPI had limited value in primary tumor detection and locoregional lymph node metastasis. RI ≥ 10% might improve the sensitivity and specificity of detection of distant metastasis
Shinya et al,[103] 2012	DTPI in patients with malignant lymphoma	Lymphoma	43	SUV_{max}, RI	SUV_{max} at second hour was significantly higher than at first hour. DTPI with semiquantitative approach might be able to accurately diagnose, stage, and predict lymphoma subtypes compared with STPI
Miyake et al,[104] 2012	Clinical value of early delayed scanning (85 min postinjection) in comparison with conventional delayed scanning (124 min postinjection) in colorectal cancer	Colorectal cancer	54	Visual, SUV_{max}	Neither 85-min nor 124-min postinjection scan improved the staging of colorectal cancer

Lee et al,[105] 2012	Relationship between DTPI and immunohistochemical factors in preoperative colorectal cancer	Colorectal cancer	47	SUV_{max}, RI	Higher RIs in patients with advanced T stage. Patients with higher levels of GLUT1 had increased RIs. Patients with increased p53 had slightly increased RIs compared with patients without increased p53. T staging was independently correlated with RI. RI has the potential to be used as a prognostic marker
Hahn et al,[57] 2012	Axillary lymph node metastasis detection in patients with breast cancer using DTPI	Breast cancer	38	SUV_{max}	The sensitivity, specificity, PPV, NPV, and accuracy for detection of axillary lymph node metastasis were not statistically significant at 2 time points
Garcia Vicente et al,[22] 2012	Biological prognostic factors and DTPI in locally advanced breast cancer	Breast cancer	36	SUV_{max}, RI	RI was superior to SUV_{max} values regarding correlation with biological parameters and can be suggested as a prognostic marker
Chang et al,[14] 2012	Correlation of DTPI with Ki-67 proliferation index in new cases of non-Hodgkin lymphoma	Lymphoma	27	SUV_{max}, RI	DTPI was shown to be feasible for measurement of tumor proliferation
Prieto et al,[106] 2011	DTPI for brain tumor identification and delineation	Brain tumor	25	SUV, tumor/normal gray matter ratio	Quantitative DTPI improves the sensitivity for detection and delineation of advanced brain tumors
Kim et al,[107] 2011	DTPI in diagnosis and prediction of incidental thyroid nodules	Thyroid nodules	50	Visual, %ΔSUV_{max}	All indices were similar in efficacy for diagnosis and prediction of malignancy

Abbreviations: %ΔSUV_{max}, percent change SUV_{max}; NPV, negative predictive value; PPV, positive predictive value; RI, retention index; SD, standard deviation; STPI, single-time-point imaging; TLR, tumor/liver uptake ratio.

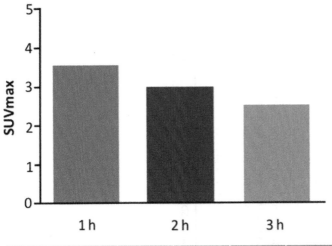

Fig. 3. Hepatic FDG uptake over time in a study including 30 patients undergoing FDG-PET at 1, 2, and 3 hours postinjection. The region of interest was placed on the dome of the liver in the right upper lobe with the largest area excluding any CT abnormalities and SUV_{max} was measured. FDG activity in the liver showed significant decrease over time. This trend was also seen with aorta blood pool. The reason for this finding might be that high levels of glucose-6-phosphatase in the liver hydrolyzed the FDG-6-phosphate and released the free FDG to the bloodstream. High FDG uptake in the liver results in suboptimal detection of primary hepatocellular carcinoma as well as metastatic lesions. Therefore, delayed FDG-PET at 3 hours with substantial washout of FDG (28.3% in this study) potentially enhances the clinical application of FDG-PET in liver malignancies and possibly other lesions.

Liver	P value	Mean of SUV difference	Mean of RI	95% CI of SUV difference	95% CI of RI
1 to 2 h	<.0004	−.1334	−.189	−.0648 to −.2021	−16.5 to −21.2
2 to 3 h	<.0001	−.22433	−.115	−.1829 to −.26577	9.652 to 13.28
1 to 3 h	<.0001	−.6679	−.283	−.5974 to −.7385	−26.07 to −30.43

1-unit increase, PFS and OS were 21.1% and 46.2%, respectively (all P<.01). This study recognized DTPI as a promising technique for prognostication of outcome in patients with lung cancer.

Role of dual-time-point imaging in lymph node staging of lung cancer

Several studies have shown the applicability of FDG-PET/CT in lymph node staging and

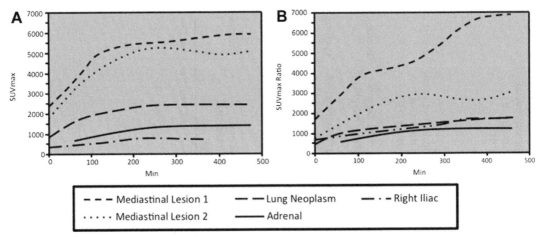

Fig. 4. The time-activity curves of malignant lesions in 3 patients with diagnosis of NSCLC undergoing whole-body FDG-PET at multiple time points from 5 minutes to 8 hours after injection of FDG. (A) Time-activity curve of malignant lesions in the mediastinum, lung, adrenal, and right iliac area represented by SUV_{max}. (B) Time-activity curve of the same lesions represented by SUV_{max} ratios with those of normal lung. These graphs show the importance of delayed imaging in detecting lesions in various sites, which may allow the accurate staging of various malignancies. Furthermore, these data reveal tumor heterogeneity of cancer at different anatomic sites. Such findings may explain the different biology as cancer spreads to other organs and the lack of response to treatment. (*Data from* Basu S, Kung J, Houseni M, et al. Temporal profile of fluorodeoxyglucose uptake in malignant lesions and normal organs over extended time periods in patients with lung carcinoma: implications for its utilization in assessing malignant lesions. Q J Nucl Med Mol Imaging 2009;53(1):9–19.)

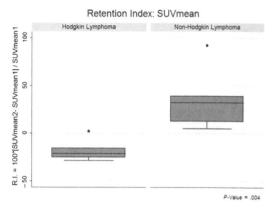

Retention Index: SUVmean

P-Value = .004

Fig. 5. Twelve patients with Hodgkin and non-Hodgkin lymphoma who were imaged at 1 and 3 hours, showing different trends over time. Although retention index (RI) in patients with Hodgkin lymphoma shows washout over time, the reverse seems to be the case with patients with non-Hodgkin lymphoma: patients with non-Hodgkin lymphoma show similar findings to patients with solid tumors and retain more FDG over time, whereas Hodgkin lymphoma, similar to other inflammatory processes, loses its activity after initial high uptake. This finding is an indication that Hodgkin lymphoma represents an inflammatory disorder, as has been speculated from other findings on clinical and histopathologic examination.

metastases to the lymph nodes.[50] DTPI has also been investigated for detection of lymph node metastasis in lung cancer in order to determine whether this technique increases the accuracy of this imaging modality. Shen and colleagues[51] in a meta-analysis assessed the diagnostic performance of FDG-PET/CT mediastinal lymph node metastasis detection in 8 studies consisting of 654 patients with NSCLC using DTPI and STPI. Despite significant heterogeneity between the studies, DTPI had overall superior performance compared with STPI for detection of mediastinal lymph nodes with regard to AUC (0.87 for DTPI and 0.83 for STPI per patient analysis, 0.93 for DTPI and 0.89 for STPI per lesion analysis) and diagnostic odds ratio (per patient analysis was 16.91; 95% CI, 6.83–41.87 for DTPI and 10.81, 95% CI, 5.48–21.33 for STPI PET/CT. Per lesion analysis was 35.4; 95% CI, 12.69–98.77 for DTPI and 21.94; 95% CI, 13.26–36.31 for STPI PET/CT).[51] The investigators concluded that further studies are needed to clarify the role of DTPI.

Kim and colleagues[52] in a study of 69 patients with NSCLC in a predominant area of pulmonary tuberculosis, performed DTPI FDG-PET/CT and found significantly higher accuracy of delayed SUV_{max} (AUC, 0.884) compared with early SUV_{max} and retention index (RI) (AUC, 0.868 and 0.717,

respectively; $P<.01$) for detection of mediastinal lymph nodes. Therefore, DTPI was considered to increase the accuracy of lymph node detection in NSCLC. Shinozaki and colleagues used DTPI for preoperative staging of 100 patients with lung cancer and noted upstaging of 10% of patients and downstaging of 5% of them using early FDG-PET/CT. Therefore, DTPI had a minor impact on the staging and management of this patient group. However, this study had a limited number of patients who had already been diagnosed with interpretations from 1 observer in 1 single center.

Breast

The most common malignancy in the women is breast cancer.[53] It is also recognized as the second leading cause of mortality in Western societies.[53] FDG-PET/CT has been shown to be a highly diagnostic imaging modality for diagnosis, staging, and selection of proper treatment in this patient group.[24,54,55] Several studies have investigated the applicability of DTPI for improvement of the results from FDG-PET/CT for diagnosis, assessment of axillary lymph nodes, and recurrence of breast cancer.[24,25,56–59] Mavi and colleagues[24] in a study of 152 patients with DTPI observed an increase in the uptake of FDG at the second time point in patients with malignant breast lesions. They also noted differences in the increase of FDG uptake, which might reflect the tumor biology.[24] In a more recent diagnostic study of breast lesions using DTPI in 59 patients at the first and third hour, Caprio and colleagues[20] noted accuracy, sensitivity, and specificity of 85%, 81%, and 100% for DTPI compared with 69%, 63%, and 100% in STPI, respectively. Staging of axillary lymph nodes is the most important factor for prognostication of patients with breast cancer. FDG-PET/CT using DTPI has been investigated for noninvasive assessment of nodal status in the axilla.[57,60] However, the sensitivity of FDG-PET/CT for detection of axillary lymph nodes is reported to be low[61] and subsequent studies showed that DTPI does not improve the performance of STPI. For example, Choi and colleagues[56] investigated 171 breast cancer cases using DTPI at 1 and 3 hours postinjection and found suboptimal and equal sensitivity and specificity (60.3% and 84.7%, respectively) at 2 time points. Based on these studies, DTPI seems to be useful for diagnosis of primary cancer but it does not improve the axillary lymph node staging. Further studies by application of novel modalities such as PET/MRI and total body FDG-PET scanning over delayed time points[62] might be able to improve the diagnosis and prognosis of breast cancer.

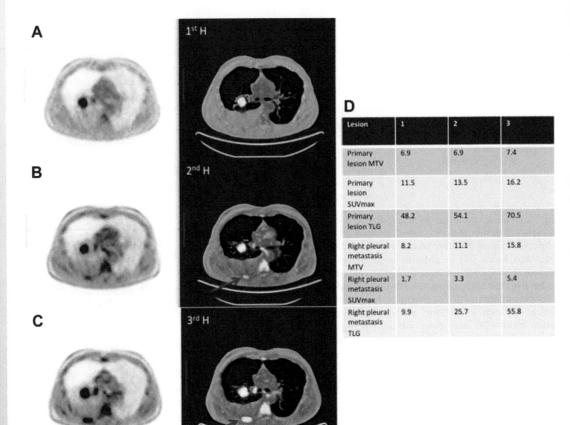

Fig. 6. Multiple-time-point FDG-PET imaging in a patient with lung cancer at the first, second, and third hours (A–C). In addition to the primary tumor and metastasis in the right hilum, a mass in the right-sided pleura, which is not visible at the first time point, becomes detectable at the delayed time points (*red arrows*). (*D*) MTV, SUV$_{max}$, and TLG of the primary and metastatic lesions of this patient.

Lesion	1	2	3
Primary lesion MTV	6.9	6.9	7.4
Primary lesion SUVmax	11.5	13.5	16.2
Primary lesion TLG	48.2	54.1	70.5
Right pleural metastasis MTV	8.2	11.1	15.8
Right pleural metastasis SUVmax	1.7	3.3	5.4
Right pleural metastasis TLG	9.9	25.7	55.8

APPLICATIONS OF DUAL-TIME-POINT IMAGING IN NONMALIGNANT DISEASES

Inflammation/Infection of the Lung

In addition to benign/malignant differentiation, DTPI has been used for diagnosis prediction of disease progression in patients with idiopathic interstitial pneumonitis (IIP).[63] Fifty patients with IIP, including 21 patients with idiopathic pulmonary fibrosis (IPF), 18 with nonspecific interstitial pneumonia (NSIP), and 11 with cryptogenic organizing pneumonia (COP), were scanned at the first and third hours after FDG injection and quantitative parameters such as mean SUV (SUV$_{mean}$) and RI were calculated and compared with pulmonary function test and imaging (CT) findings. The first time point SUV for COP (2.47 ± 0.74) was higher than the SUV of IPF (0.99 ± 0.29; P = .0002) and NSIP at the first time point (1.22 ± 0.44; P = .0025). The cutoff value of 1.5 had sensitivity, specificity, and accuracy of 90.9, 94.3%, and 93.5% for distinguishing COP from

IPF and NSIP. An RI cutoff value of 0% was able to distinguish progressive types of IIP from stable IIPs with sensitivity, specificity, and accuracy of 95.5, 100%, and 97.8%, respectively.

Involvement of the lungs happens in more than 90% of patients with sarcoidosis.[64] Most of these cases resolve with time but some patients develop persistent disease, which leads to fibrosis and might be fatal.[65] Therefore, it is important to have a prognostic measure for lung involvement in this group of patients. DTPI has been used for assessment of lung involvement in patients with sarcoidosis.[66] In this study, 21 sarcoidosis patients were undergone FDG-PET/CT at two time points (1 and 3 hours after FDG injection). SUV$_{mean}$ and RI were calculated and compared with CT imaging taken a year later. RI was higher in the group of patients with increased or unchanged pulmonary lesions based on follow-up CT (21.3% ± 9.6%) compared with the patients with improved lesions (−9.2% ± 28.6%;

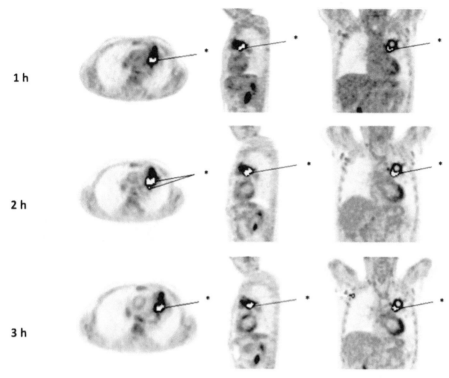

Left Lung Tumor (*)	MTV	SUVmax	SUVmean	pvcSUVmean	TLG	pvcTLG
1 h	7.8	18.3	10.9	18.4	85.1	144.1
2 h	7.9 (1.28%)	23.6 (28.96%)	14.2 (30.28%)	23.4 (27.17%)	111.8 (31.37%)	184.8 (28.24%)
3 h	8.4 (7.69%)	26.7 (45.9%)	15.7 (44.04%)	26 (41.3%)	132.5 (55.7%)	218.8 (51.84%)

Fig. 7. Multiple-time-point FDG-PET of a patient with left upper lobe malignancy. Sagittal, axial, and coronal PET scans of the patient at the first, second, and third hours are shown in the top 3 rows. The left upper lobe tumor (*asterisks*) is segmented using a commercial tool and PET parameters including MTV, TLG, SUV_{max}, SUV_{mean}, pvcSUVmean, and pvcTLG are quantified in the bottom chart. There is an increasing trend of FDG uptake in various parameters over time.

$P<.01$). In addition, serum soluble interleukin-2, which is a marker of the disease activity, was significantly correlated with RI.

One of the challenging topics in medical imaging is diagnosis of TB and differentiation of active from inactive disease, and also active TB from malignant lesions.[67] FDG-PET/CT is able to detect pulmonary and extrapulmonary TB simultaneously and is widely used in the clinic for diagnosis, staging, and treatment assessment of TB.[67] However, based on the results from several clinical trials,[17,68–70] because of the significant overlap between SUV values of active TB lesions and malignant lesion, STPI and DTPI are limited in assessment of patients with TB.[71–73] Assessment of treatment response is the most important

application of DTPI of FDG-PET/CT in the clinic because of the rapid change in the molecular characteristics of the lesions compared with structural changes after therapy, especially in the multidrug-resistant TB–endemic areas of developing countries.[67,74–77]

Atherosclerosis

It has been shown that atherosclerotic plaques are best visualized with delayed-time-point FDG-PET imaging.[28,78,79] In one study,[28] 15 patients received triple-time-point (1, 2, and 3 hours after FDG administration) FDG-PET/CT and aortic and carotid FDG uptake corresponding with atherosclerosis based on the previous studies[80,81] was

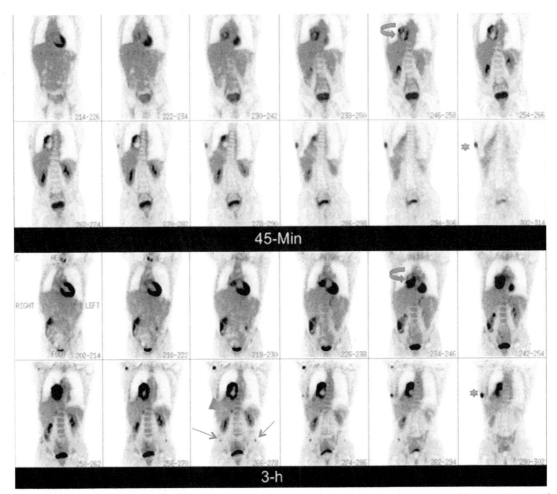

Fig. 8. Coronal FDG-PET images at 45 minutes and 3 hours of a patient with lung cancer. In addition to increased FDG uptake in the primary lung lesion in the right hilar region (*curved arrow*) and right chest wall (*star*), new lesions appear on the delayed-time-point images at the iliac bones of both sides (*arrows*) and the right adrenal gland (*arrowhead*).

qualitatively and semiquantitatively measured. The qualitative assessment showed improvement of plaque visualization on delayed times. From the first hour to the third hour the target/background ratio (TBR) in the aorta and carotid increased from 1.05 and 0.88 to 1.57 and 1.61, respectively. Another study[29] designed to correlate FDG uptake at 2 time points (90 and 180 minutes) with 10-year risk for fatal cardiovascular disease in 40 patients, found significant increase in the carotid blood pool corrected SUV_{max} ($cSUV_{max}$; 23%; $P<.0001$) and TBR (20%; $P<.0001$), aortic $cSUV_{max}$ (14%; $P<.0001$) and TBR (20%; $P<.0001$) over time. At the first time point, there was no correlation with 10-year risk of cardiovascular disease, whereas the second time point had a significant correlation ($cSUV_{max}$ of the carotid arteries $\tau = 0.25$, $P = .045$ and aorta $\tau = 0.33$, $P = .008$). Bucerius and colleagues[79] evaluated the impact of different parameters, including circulation time of radiotracer, injected dose, and blood glucose, in the aorta and carotid arteries of 195 scans using multivariate regression analyses. The circulation time of 2.5 hours and glucose levels less than 7.0 mmol/L had favorable relationships between arterial and blood pool FDG uptake.

These findings support the theory of improvement in the contrast between target tissues regardless of their underlying disease process (eg, cancer, inflammation), and increase in the sensitivity of FDG-PET in detecting various abnormalities in many organs over time with decline in the background blood pool (see **Fig. 1**).

Brown Fat

Human adipose tissue consists of 2 main types: brown and white.[82] The main function of white fat

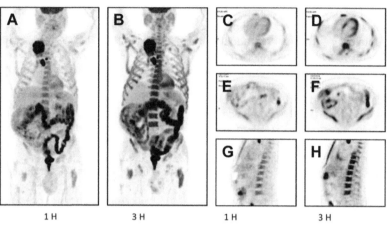

| 1 H | 3 H | 1 H | 3 H |

Fig. 9. Delayed-time-point imaging revealing new lesions in bone marrow. A 69-year old man with a lung mass underwent multiple-time-point FDG-PET/CT imaging for diagnostic evaluation. The initial PET imaging (performed at 1 hour after tracer injection) revealed equivocal bone marrow uptake in the right iliac bone and proximal femurs in addition to lung and mediastinal lesions. However, the 3-hour delayed PET imaging showed widespread bone marrow metastases. Biopsies of the right lung mass and right iliac bone marrow were later performed and revealed a poorly differentiated squamous cell carcinoma at both sites. (*A, B:* maximum intensity projection view of the patient at 1st and 3rd hours, respectively; *C, E, G:* Transaxial and sagittal view of the same patient at 1-hour; *D, F, H:* Transaxial and sagittal view of the same patient at 3-hour.)

is protection, whereas brown fat generates heat. Brown fat has many mitochondria.[82] Although they have a wide distribution and variable degrees of FDG uptake, they are mostly bilateral, symmetric, and elongated, and are visible in the supraclavicular, mediastinal, paravertebral, and perirenal regions.[83] One of the sources of false-positive results in FDG-PET imaging is the presence of metabolically active brown adipose tissue, which resembles malignant lesions.[82–84] Various studies have shown diverse patterns of FDG uptake in STPI and DTPI of brown fat,[82,83] which makes it difficult to distinguish malignant lesions from brown fat tissue.

Crohn Disease

Crohn disease (CD) is inflammatory disease of the gastrointestinal system with unknown cause, which presents with lesions in the mucosa and clinical symptoms such as abdominal pain, weight loss, and diarrhea.[85] Quantitative FDG-PET/CT indices have been correlated with clinical and pathologic findings.[85] In addition, preliminary results[86] suggest that DTPI is able to predict the potential response to the treatment of CD with anti–tumor necrosis factor. Differences between global CD activity and RI before and after treatment were quantified. Treatment response was correlated with pretreatment RI ($r = 0.76$; $P = .01$), which suggests this biomarker as a potent predictor of treatment response.

In summary, there is a general consensus (even in the studies that did not show diagnostic value for DTPI) about the decrease in the background activity and increase in the SUV values in tumors in delayed-time-point imaging and DTPI, and that this improves the quality of the image[2] compared with the 60-minute imaging, which might not be sufficient. This ability might enable clinicians to improve the accuracy of the PET imaging to an extent that albeit may become possible to detect subtle metastases in patients with cancer in the near future.[62] At present, the best approach for achieving the best clinical performance seems to be selective use of DTPI in the clinic.[2] Further studies with large sample size, meta-analyses, and systematic reviews are needed to determine the definitive value of DTPI and delayed-time-point imaging in the clinic.

CHALLENGES, SUMMARY, AND FUTURE DIRECTIONS

Many studies have shown improvement in the diagnostic/prognostic accuracy of using DTPI. Even the studies that did not show this improvement, at least showed similar performance for DTPI compared with STPI.[2] However, the utility of DTPI and RI in clinical settings has faced some limitations, which prevents its application on a routine basis.[2] Some studies have shown some of these limitations. For example, differentiation between malignant and inflammatory lesions was not consistently successful using DTPI because some studies have shown nonspecificity in lung and mediastinal lesions and lung nodules with low FDG uptake.[42,66,68,69,87–89] In addition, acute infectious and noninfectious inflammatory lesions, specifically granulomatous lesions, show a pattern similar to the malignant lesions[90,91] and therefore DTPI is not considered to be superior to STPI in the areas with high prevalence of sarcoidosis and in tuberculosis (TB)-endemic areas.[42,66,68,69,88,89,92] However, DTPI is still a useful option for differentiation of inactive granulomatous or chronic inflammatory lesions from malignancy because of difference in the biological behavior of the cells involved in the chronic versus acute inflammation.[2]

REFERENCES

1. Hess S, Blomberg BA, Zhu HJ, et al. The pivotal role of FDG-PET/CT in modern medicine. Acad Radiol 2014;21(2):232–49.
2. Cheng G, Torigian DA, Zhuang H, et al. When should we recommend use of dual time-point and delayed time-point imaging techniques in FDG PET? Eur J Nucl Med Mol Imaging 2013;40(5):779–87.
3. Hustinx R, Smith RJ, Benard F, et al. Dual time point fluorine-18 fluorodeoxyglucose positron emission tomography: a potential method to differentiate malignancy from inflammation and normal tissue in the head and neck. Eur J Nucl Med 1999;26(10):1345–8.
4. Zhuang H, Pourdehnad M, Lambright ES, et al. Dual time point 18F-FDG PET imaging for differentiating malignant from inflammatory processes. J Nucl Med 2001;42(9):1412–7.
5. Matthies A, Hickeson M, Cuchiara A, et al. Dual time point 18F-FDG PET for the evaluation of pulmonary nodules. J Nucl Med 2002;43(7):871–5.
6. Higashi T, Saga T, Nakamoto Y, et al. Relationship between retention index in dual-phase (18)F-FDG PET, and hexokinase-II and glucose transporter-1 expression in pancreatic cancer. J Nucl Med 2002;43(2):173–80.
7. Basu S, Kwee TC, Surti S, et al. Fundamentals of PET and PET/CT imaging. Ann N Y Acad Sci 2011;1228:1–18.
8. Nelson CA, Wang JQ, Leav I, et al. The interaction among glucose transport, hexokinase, and glucose-6-phosphatase with respect to 3H-2-deoxyglucose retention in murine tumor models. Nucl Med Biol 1996;23(4):533–41.
9. Suzuki S, Toyota T, Suzuki H, et al. Partial purification from human mononuclear cells and placental plasma membranes of an insulin mediator which stimulates pyruvate dehydrogenase and

10. suppresses glucose-6-phosphatase. Arch Biochem Biophys 1984;235(2):418–26.
10. Strauss LG. Fluorine-18 deoxyglucose and false-positive results: a major problem in the diagnostics of oncological patients. Eur J Nucl Med 1996;23(10):1409–15.
11. Cook GJ, Maisey MN, Fogelman I. Normal variants, artefacts and interpretative pitfalls in PET imaging with 18-fluoro-2-deoxyglucose and carbon-11 methionine. Eur J Nucl Med 1999;26(10):1363–78.
12. Zhuang H, Duarte PS, Pourdehand M, et al. Exclusion of chronic osteomyelitis with F-18 fluorodeoxyglucose positron emission tomographic imaging. Clin Nucl Med 2000;25(4):281–4.
13. Alkhawaldeh K, Bural G, Kumar R, et al. Impact of dual-time-point (18)F-FDG PET imaging and partial volume correction in the assessment of solitary pulmonary nodules. Eur J Nucl Med Mol Imaging 2008;35(2):246–52.
14. Chang CC, Cho SF, Chen YW, et al. SUV on dual-phase FDG PET/CT correlates with the Ki-67 proliferation index in patients with newly diagnosed non-Hodgkin lymphoma. Clin Nucl Med 2012;37(8):e189–95.
15. Barger RL Jr, Nandalur KR. Diagnostic performance of dual-time 18F-FDG PET in the diagnosis of pulmonary nodules: a meta-analysis. Acad Radiol 2012;19(2):153–8.
16. Cheng G, Cho SF, Chen YW, et al. Serial changes of FDG uptake and diagnosis of suspected lung malignancy: a lesion-based analysis. Clin Nucl Med 2014;39(2):147–55.
17. Kaneko K, Sadashima E, Irie K, et al. Assessment of FDG retention differences between the FDG-avid benign pulmonary lesion and primary lung cancer using dual-time-point FDG-PET imaging. Ann Nucl Med 2013;27(4):392–9.
18. Khan AN, Al-Jahdali H. Value of delayed 18F-FDG PET in the diagnosis of solitary pulmonary nodule. J Thorac Dis 2013;5(3):373–4.
19. Xiu Y, Bhutani C, Dhurairaj T, et al. Dual-time point FDG PET imaging in the evaluation of pulmonary nodules with minimally increased metabolic activity. Clin Nucl Med 2007;32(2):101–5.
20. Caprio MG, Cangiano A, Imbriaco M, et al. Dual-time-point [18F]-FDG PET/CT in the diagnostic evaluation of suspicious breast lesions. Radiol Med 2010;115(2):215–24.
21. Garcia Vicente AM, Soriano Castrejón A, Cruz Mora MÁ, et al. Dual time point 2-deoxy-2-[18F] fluoro-D-glucose PET/CT: nodal staging in locally advanced breast cancer. Rev Esp Med Nucl Imagen Mol 2014;33(1):1–5.
22. Garcia Vicente AM, Soriano Castrejón A, Relea Calatayud F, et al. 18F-FDG semi-quantitative parameters and biological prognostic factors in

locally advanced breast cancer. Rev Esp Med Nucl Imagen Mol 2012;31(6):308–14.

23. Kumar R, Loving VA, Chauhan A, et al. Potential of dual-time-point imaging to improve breast cancer diagnosis with (18)F-FDG PET. J Nucl Med 2005; 46(11):1819–24.

24. Mavi A, Urhan M, Yu JQ, et al. Dual time point 18F-FDG PET imaging detects breast cancer with high sensitivity and correlates well with histologic subtypes. J Nucl Med 2006;47(9):1440–6.

25. Zytoon AA, Murakami K, El-Kholy MR, et al. Dual time point FDG-PET/CT imaging. Potential tool for diagnosis of breast cancer. Clin Radiol 2008; 63(11):1213–27.

26. Abgral R, Le Roux PY, Rousset J, et al. Prognostic value of dual-time-point 18F-FDG PET-CT imaging in patients with head and neck squamous cell carcinoma. Nucl Med Commun 2013; 34(6):551–6.

27. Lyshchik A, Higashi T, Nakamoto Y, et al. Dual-phase 18F-fluoro-2-deoxy-D-glucose positron emission tomography as a prognostic parameter in patients with pancreatic cancer. Eur J Nucl Med Mol Imaging 2005;32(4):389–97.

28. Blomberg BA, Akers SR, Saboury B, et al. Delayed time-point 18F-FDG PET CT imaging enhances assessment of atherosclerotic plaque inflammation. Nucl Med Commun 2013;34(9):860–7.

29. Blomberg BA, Thomassen A, Takx RA, et al. Delayed (1)(8)F-fluorodeoxyglucose PET/CT imaging improves quantitation of atherosclerotic plaque inflammation: results from the CAMONA study. J Nucl Cardiol 2014;21(3):588–97.

30. Chirindel A, Chaudhry M, Blakeley JO, et al. 18F-FDG PET/CT qualitative and quantitative evaluation in NF1 patients for detection of malignant transformation - comparison of early to delayed imaging with and without liver activity normalization. J Nucl Med 2015;56(3):379–85.

31. Salavati A, Saboury B, Alavi A. Comment on: "Tumor aggressiveness and patient outcome in cancer of the pancreas assessed by dynamic 18F-FDG PET/CT". J Nucl Med 2014;55(2):350–1.

32. Whaley JT, Fernandes AT, Sackmann R, et al. Clinical utility of integrated positron emission tomography/computed tomography imaging in the clinical management and radiation treatment planning of locally advanced rectal cancer. Pract Radiat Oncol 2014;4(4):226–32.

33. Houshmand S, Salavati A, Basu S, et al. The role of dual and multiple time point imaging of FDG uptake in both normal and disease states. Clin Transl Imaging 2014;2(4):281–93.

34. Basu S, Zaidi H, Houseni M, et al. Novel quantitative techniques for assessing regional and global function and structure based on modern imaging modalities: implications for normal variation, aging and diseased states. Semin Nucl Med 2007; 37(3):223–39.

35. Basu S, Alavi A. Partial volume correction of standardized uptake values and the dual time point in FDG-PET imaging: should these be routinely employed in assessing patients with cancer? Eur J Nucl Med Mol Imaging 2007; 34(10):1527–9.

36. Cheng G, Alavi A, Lim E, et al. Dynamic changes of FDG uptake and clearance in normal tissues. Mol Imaging Biol 2013;15(3):345–52.

37. Cheng G, Alavi A, Lee NJ, et al. Differential background clearance of fluorodeoxyglucose activity in normal tissues and its clinical significance. PET Clinics 2014;9(2):209–16.

38. Choi GG, Han Y, Weston B, et al. Metabolic effects of pulmonary obstruction on myocardial functioning: a pilot study using multiple time-point 18F-FDG-PET imaging. Nucl Med Commun 2015; 36(1):78–83.

39. Basu S, Kung J, Houseni M, et al. Temporal profile of fluorodeoxyglucose uptake in malignant lesions and normal organs over extended time periods in patients with lung carcinoma: implications for its utilization in assessing malignant lesions. Q J Nucl Med Mol Imaging 2009;53(1):9–19.

40. Higgins GA, Shields TW, Keehn RJ. The solitary pulmonary nodule. Ten-year follow-up of Veterans Administration-Armed Forces Cooperative Study. Arch Surg 1975;110(5):570–5.

41. Lillington GA, Caskey CI. Evaluation and management of solitary and multiple pulmonary nodules. Clin Chest Med 1993;14(1):111–9.

42. Laffon E, de Clermont H, Begueret H, et al. Assessment of dual-time-point 18F-FDG-PET imaging for pulmonary lesions. Nucl Med Commun 2009; 30(6):455–61.

43. Lin YY, Chen JH, Ding HJ, et al. Potential value of dual-time-point (1)(8)F-FDG PET compared with initial single-time-point imaging in differentiating malignant from benign pulmonary nodules: a systematic review and meta-analysis. Nucl Med Commun 2012;33(10):1011–8.

44. Zhang L, Wang Y, Lei J, et al. Dual time point 18FDG-PET/CT versus single time point 18FDG-PET/CT for the differential diagnosis of pulmonary nodules: a meta-analysis. Acta Radiol 2013;54(7): 770–7.

45. Gould MK, Maclean CC, Kuschner WG, et al. Accuracy of positron emission tomography for diagnosis of pulmonary nodules and mass lesions: a meta-analysis. JAMA 2001;285(7):914–24.

46. Chen HH, Lee BF, Su WC, et al. The increment in standardized uptake value determined using dual-phase 18F-FDG PET is a promising prognostic factor in non-small-cell lung cancer. Eur J Nucl Med Mol Imaging 2013;40(10):1478–85.

47. Houseni M, Chamroonrat W, Zhuang J, et al. Prognostic implication of dual-phase PET in adenocarcinoma of the lung. J Nucl Med 2010; 51(4):535–42.

48. Satoh Y, Nambu A, Onishi H, et al. Value of dual time point F-18 FDG-PET/CT imaging for the evaluation of prognosis and risk factors for recurrence in patients with stage I non-small cell lung cancer treated with stereotactic body radiation therapy. Eur J Radiol 2012;81(11):3530–4.

49. Kim SJ, Kim YK, Kim IJ, et al. Limited prognostic value of dual time point F-18 FDG PET/CT in patients with early stage (stage I & II) non-small cell lung cancer (NSCLC). Radiother Oncol 2011; 98(1):105–8.

50. Kim YK, Lee KS, Kim BT, et al. Mediastinal nodal staging of nonsmall cell lung cancer using integrated 18F-FDG PET/CT in a tuberculosis-endemic country: diagnostic efficacy in 674 patients. Cancer 2007;109(6):1068–77.

51. Shen G, Hu S, Deng H, et al. Diagnostic value of dual time-point 18 F-FDG PET/CT versus single time-point imaging for detection of mediastinal nodal metastasis in non-small cell lung cancer patients: a meta-analysis. Acta Radiol 2014;56(6):681–7.

52. Kim DW, Kim WH, Kim CG. Dual-time-point FDG PET/CT: is it useful for lymph node staging in patients with non-small-cell lung cancer? Nucl Med Mol Imaging 2012;46(3):196–200.

53. Siegel R, DeSantis C, Virgo K, et al. Cancer treatment and survivorship statistics, 2012. CA Cancer J Clin 2012;62(4):220–41.

54. Heusner TA, Freudenberg LS, Kuehl H, et al. Whole-body PET/CT-mammography for staging breast cancer: initial results. Br J Radiol 2008; 81(969):743–8.

55. Heusner TA, Kuemmel S, Umutlu L, et al. Breast cancer staging in a single session: whole-body PET/CT mammography. J Nucl Med 2008;49(8): 1215–22.

56. Choi WH, Yoo IR, O JH, et al. The value of dual-time-point 18F-FDG PET/CT for identifying axillary lymph node metastasis in breast cancer patients. Br J Radiol 2011;84(1003):593–9.

57. Hahn S, Hecktor J, Grabellus F, et al. Diagnostic accuracy of dual-time-point 18F-FDG PET/CT for the detection of axillary lymph node metastases in breast cancer patients. Acta Radiol 2012;53(5): 518–23.

58. Matthiessen LW, Johannesen HH, Skougaard K, et al. Dual time point imaging fluorine-18 flourodeoxyglucose positron emission tomography for evaluation of large loco-regional recurrences of breast cancer treated with electrochemotherapy. Radiol Oncol 2013;47(4):358–65.

59. Zytoon AA, Murakami K, El-Kholy MR, et al. Breast cancer with low FDG uptake: characterization by means of dual-time point FDG-PET/CT. Eur J Radiol 2009;70(3):530–8.

60. Choi EK, Yoo IeR, Kim SH, et al. The clinical value of dual-time point 18F-FDG PET/CT for differentiating extrahepatic cholangiocarcinoma from benign disease. Clin Nucl Med 2013;38(3): e106–11.

61. Crippa F, Gerali A, Alessi A, et al. FDG-PET for axillary lymph node staging in primary breast cancer. Eur J Nucl Med Mol Imaging 2004;31(Suppl 1): S97–102.

62. Price PM, Badawi RD, Cherry SR, et al. Ultra staging to unmask the prescribing of adjuvant therapy in cancer patients: the future opportunity to image micrometastases using total-body 18F-FDG PET scanning. J Nucl Med 2014;55(4): 696–7.

63. Umeda Y, Demura Y, Ishizaki T, et al. Dual-time-point 18F-FDG PET imaging for diagnosis of disease type and disease activity in patients with idiopathic interstitial pneumonia. Eur J Nucl Med Mol Imaging 2009;36(7):1121–30.

64. Hunninghake GW, Costabel U, Ando M, et al. ATS/ ERS/WASOG statement on sarcoidosis. American Thoracic Society/European Respiratory Society/ World Association of Sarcoidosis and other Granulomatous Disorders. Sarcoidosis Vasc Diffuse Lung Dis 1999;16(2):149–73.

65. NIH conference. Pulmonary sarcoidosis: a disease characterized and perpetuated by activated lung T-lymphocytes. Ann Intern Med 1981;94(1): 73–94.

66. Umeda Y, Demura Y, Morikawa M, et al. Prognostic value of dual-time-point 18F-fluorodeoxyglucose positron emission tomography in patients with pulmonary sarcoidosis. Respirology 2011;16(4): 713–20.

67. Vorster M, Sathekge MM, Bomanji J. Advances in imaging of tuberculosis: the role of (1)(8)F-FDG PET and PET/CT. Curr Opin Pulm Med 2014; 20(3):287–93.

68. Chen C-J, Lee BF, Yao WJ, et al. Dual-phase 18F-FDG PET in the diagnosis of pulmonary nodules with an initial standard uptake value less than 2.5. AJR Am J Roentgenol 2008;191(2):475–9.

69. Sathekge MM, Maes A, Pottel H, et al. Dual time-point FDG PET-CT for differentiating benign from malignant solitary pulmonary nodules in a TB endemic area. S Afr Med J 2010;100(9):598–601.

70. Kim IJ, Lee JS, Kim SJ, et al. Double-phase 18F-FDG PET-CT for determination of pulmonary tuberculoma activity. Eur J Nucl Med Mol Imaging 2008; 35(4):808–14.

71. Chang JM, Lee HJ, Goo JM, et al. False positive and false negative FDG-PET scans in various thoracic diseases. Korean J Radiol 2006;7(1): 57–69.

72. Brown RS, Leung JY, Fisher SJ, et al. Intratumoral distribution of tritiated fluorodeoxyglucose in breast carcinoma: I. Are inflammatory cells important? J Nucl Med 1995;36(10):1854–61.

73. Bakheet SM, Powe J. Benign causes of 18-FDG uptake on whole body imaging. Semin Nucl Med 1998;28(4):352–8.

74. Sathekge M, Maes A, Van de Wiele C. FDG-PET imaging in HIV infection and tuberculosis. Semin Nucl Med 2013;43(5):349–66.

75. Hofmeyr A, Lau WF, Slavin MA. *Mycobacterium tuberculosis* infection in patients with cancer, the role of 18-fluorodeoxyglucose positron emission tomography for diagnosis and monitoring treatment response. Tuberculosis (Edinb) 2007;87(5):459–63.

76. Park IN, Ryu JS, Shim TS. Evaluation of therapeutic response of tuberculoma using F-18 FDG positron emission tomography. Clin Nucl Med 2008;33(1):1–3.

77. Sathekge M, Maes A, Kgomo M, et al. Use of 18F-FDG PET to predict response to first-line tuberculostatics in HIV-associated tuberculosis. J Nucl Med 2011;52(6):880–5.

78. Gholami S, Salavati A, Houshmand S, et al. Assessment of atherosclerosis in large vessel walls: a comprehensive review of FDG-PET/CT image acquisition protocols and methods for uptake quantification. J Nucl Cardiol 2015;22(3):468–79.

79. Bucerius J, Mani V, Moncrieff C, et al. Optimizing 18F-FDG PET/CT imaging of vessel wall inflammation: the impact of 18F-FDG circulation time, injected dose, uptake parameters, and fasting blood glucose levels. Eur J Nucl Med Mol Imaging 2014;41(2):369–83.

80. Yun M, Jang S, Cucchiara A, et al. 18F FDG uptake in the large arteries: a correlation study with the atherogenic risk factors. Semin Nucl Med 2002;32(1):70–6.

81. Yun M, Yeh D, Araujo LI, et al. F-18 FDG uptake in the large arteries: a new observation. Clin Nucl Med 2001;26(4):314–9.

82. Hairil Rashmizal AR, Noraini AR, Rossetti C, et al. Brown fat uptake of 18F-FDG on dual time point PET/CT imaging. Singapore Med J 2010;51(2):e37–9.

83. Alkhawaldeh K, Alavi A. Quantitative assessment of FDG uptake in brown fat using standardized uptake value and dual-time-point scanning. Clin Nucl Med 2008;33(10):663–7.

84. Basu S, Alavi A. Optimizing interventions for preventing uptake in the brown adipose tissue in FDG-PET. Eur J Nucl Med Mol Imaging 2008;35(8):1421–3.

85. Saboury B, Salavati A, Brothers A, et al. FDG PET/CT in Crohn's disease: correlation of quantitative FDG PET/CT parameters with clinical and endoscopic surrogate markers of disease activity. Eur J Nucl Med Mol Imaging 2014;41(4):605–14.

86. Saboury B, Salavati A, Sanz-Viedma S, et al. Pre-treatment dual-time-point FDG-PET/CT imaging may predict response in patients with Crohn's disease. J Nucl Med Meeting Abstracts 2013;54(2_MeetingAbstracts):587.

87. Cloran FJ, Banks KP, Song WS, et al. Limitations of dual time point PET in the assessment of lung nodules with low FDG avidity. Lung Cancer 2010;68(1):66–71.

88. Li M, Wu N, Liu Y, et al. Regional nodal staging with 18F-FDG PET-CT in non-small cell lung cancer: additional diagnostic value of CT attenuation and dual-time-point imaging. Eur J Radiol 2012;81(8):1886–90.

89. Zheng Z, Pan Y, Guo F, et al. Multimodality FDG PET/CT appearance of pulmonary tuberculoma mimicking lung cancer and pathologic correlation in a tuberculosis-endemic country. South Med J 2011;104(6):440–5.

90. Kok PJ, van Eerd JE, Boerman OC, et al. Bio-distribution and imaging of FDG in rats with LS174T carcinoma xenografts and focal *Escherichia coli* infection. Cancer Biother Radiopharm 2005;20(3):310–5.

91. Makinen TJ, Lankinen P, Pöyhönen T, et al. Comparison of 18F-FDG and 68Ga PET imaging in the assessment of experimental osteomyelitis due to *Staphylococcus aureus*. Eur J Nucl Med Mol Imaging 2005;32(11):1259–68.

92. Yen RF, Chen KC, Lee JM, et al. 18F-FDG PET for the lymph node staging of non-small cell lung cancer in a tuberculosis-endemic country: is dual time point imaging worth the effort? Eur J Nucl Med Mol Imaging 2008;35(7):1305–15.

93. Shinozaki T, Utano K, Fujii H, et al. Routine use of dual time F-FDG PET for staging of preoperative lung cancer: does it affect clinical management? Jpn J Radiol 2014;32(8):476–81.

94. Lee S, Park T, Park S, et al. The clinical role of dual-time-point (18)F-FDG PET/CT in differential diagnosis of the thyroid incidentaloma. Nucl Med Mol Imaging 2014;48(2):121–9.

95. Kim SJ, Kim YK, Kim IJ, et al. Limited predictive value of dual-time-point F-18 FDG PET/CT for evaluation of pathologic N1 status in NSCLC patients. Clin Nucl Med 2011;36(6):434–9.

96. Macdonald K, Searle J, Lyburn I. The role of dual time point FDG PET imaging in the evaluation of solitary pulmonary nodules with an initial standard uptake value less than 2.5. Clin Radiol 2011;66(3):244–50.

97. Lee JW, Kim SK, Lee SM, et al. Detection of hepatic metastases using dual-time-point FDG PET/CT

scans in patients with colorectal cancer. Mol Imaging Biol 2011;13(3):565–72.

98. Yoon HJ, Kim SK, Kim TS, et al. New application of dual point 18F-FDG PET/CT in the evaluation of neoadjuvant chemoradiation response of locally advanced rectal cancer. Clin Nucl Med 2013; 38(1):7–12.

99. Toriihara A, Nakamura S, Kubota K, et al. Can dual-time-point 18F-FDG PET/CT differentiate malignant salivary gland tumors from benign tumors? AJR Am J Roentgenol 2013;201(3):639–44.

100. Nakayama M, Okizaki A, Ishitoya S, et al. Dual-time-point F-18 FDG PET/CT imaging for differentiating the lymph nodes between malignant lymphoma and benign lesions. Ann Nucl Med 2013;27(2):163–9.

101. Costantini DL, Vali R, Chan J, et al. Dual-time-point FDG PET/CT for the evaluation of pediatric tumors. AJR Am J Roentgenol 2013;200(2):408–13.

102. Shum WY, Hsieh TC, Yeh JJ, et al. Clinical usefulness of dual-time FDG PET-CT in assessment of esophageal squamous cell carcinoma. Eur J Radiol 2012;81(5):1024–8.

103. Shinya T, Fujii S, Asakura S, et al. Dual-time-point F-18 FDG PET/CT for evaluation in patients with malignant lymphoma. Ann Nucl Med 2012;26(8): 616–21.

104. Miyake KK, Nakamoto Y, Togashi K. Dual-time-point 18F-FDG PET/CT in patients with colorectal cancer: clinical value of early delayed scanning. Ann Nucl Med 2012;26(6):492–500.

105. Lee JH, Lee WA, Park SG, et al. Relationship between dual-time point FDG PET and immunohistochemical parameters in preoperative colorectal cancer: preliminary study. Nucl Med Mol Imaging 2012;46(1):48–56.

106. Prieto E, Martí-Climent JM, Domínguez-Prado I, et al. Voxel-based analysis of dual-time-point 18F-FDG PET images for brain tumor identification and delineation. J Nucl Med 2011;52(6): 865–72.

107. Kim SJ, Kim BH, Jeon YK, et al. Limited diagnostic and predictive values of dual-time-point 18F FDG PET/CT for differentiation of incidentally detected thyroid nodules. Ann Nucl Med 2011; 25(5):347–53.

Contrast Media in PET/ Computed Tomography Imaging

Varun Singh Dhull, MBBS, MD[a],*, Neelima Rana, MBBS, MD[b],
Aftab Hasan Nazar, MBBS, MD[a]

KEYWORDS

- FDG PET/CT • Intravenous contrast • Oral contrast • Diuretic PET/CT • PET/CT enteroclysis

KEY POINTS

- Contrast agents are usually given orally or intravenously.
- Intravenous contrast agents are usually iodine based (ionic and nonionic), and oral contrast agents can be grouped into positive and negative agents.
- State-of-the-art diagnostic PET/computed tomography (CT) scan with intravenous or oral contrast gives excellent anatomic details as well as information on tumor vascularization and reduces the need for additional contrast-enhanced diagnostic imaging modalities.
- Contrast agents (especially positive oral contrast agents) in PET/CT may lead to overestimation of PET attenuation factors; however, this increase/overestimation of standardized uptake value is clinically insignificant.
- Use of positive oral contrast agents should be limited to patients in whom the pathologic abnormality or site of suspected disease is in the gastrointestinal tract or abdomen.

INTRODUCTION

Contrast agents, also called contrast materials or contrast media, are now an integral part of the diagnostic radiology. They improve the visibility of internal body structures imaged by radiographs, ultrasonography, computed tomography (CT), and magnetic resonance (MR) imaging scans. They make certain structures or tissues in the body appear in a different way and thus help in distinguishing a contrast-enhanced area of the body from the surrounding tissue.

As compared with earlier times, they are now much safer and better tolerated. However, adverse reactions of varying degrees can still occur, and one needs to be aware of the basic characteristics, indications, and side effects of these contrast agents so that, in case of emergency, prompt measures can be taken.[1]

Dual-modality 18F-fluorodeoxyglucose ([18F-FDG]) PET/CT combines the advantages of the metabolic information provided by PET and the spatial and contrast resolution of CT.[2,3] FDG PET/CT has stood the test of the time and has been shown to be useful for the evaluation of various malignancies.[4,5] It has an edge over the stand-alone CT and has been shown to improve the diagnostic accuracy in various malignant disorders.[6]

Now, do we need contrast-enhanced PET/CT (PET/CECT) or is the low-dose, non-contrast-enhanced PET/CT sufficient? The question has been raised time and again, and the debate is

The authors have nothing to disclose.
[a] Department of Nuclear Medicine, All India Institute of Medical Sciences, New Delhi, India; [b] Department of Radiodiagnosis, MS Ramaiah Medical College, Bengaluru, Karnataka, India
* Corresponding author. Room No. 54, Department of Nuclear Medicine, All India Institute of Medical Sciences, Ansari Nagar, New Delhi 110029, India.
E-mail address: drvarundhull@gmail.com

PET Clin 11 (2016) 85–94
http://dx.doi.org/10.1016/j.cpet.2015.07.007
1556-8598/16/$ – see front matter © 2016 Elsevier Inc. All rights reserved.

endless.[7-9] Some favor the use of low-dose non-contrast CT that serves the purpose of simple anatomic correlation with PET and attenuation correction of PET images, reduces acquisition time, reduces radiation burden, and prevents attenuation-related artifacts by the contrast media that may lead to overestimation of standardized uptake value (SUV).[10,11] However, another school of thought supports the use of diagnostic CECT because it improves lesion detection and characterization that reduces equivocal findings and has an immediate clinical relevance. Although radiation burden is increased, the clinical benefit to the patient outweighs it.[12,13] In this review, various such issues related to the use of contrast agents and special techniques of clinical interest based on their utility in dual-modality PET/CT are addressed.

TYPES OF CONTRAST AGENTS
Intravenous Contrast Agents

Studies have shown that the addition of CECT to PET instead of noncontrast CT helps in better differentiation of abnormal tissue from the surrounding normal tissue based on the differences in contrast enhancement (**Figs. 1–4**), improving the diagnostic accuracy and leading to fewer equivocal interpretations.[14] In the past decade, as more and more dedicated PET/CT systems have been installed in various countries, many studies describing the clinical utility of iodine-based contrast material for PET/CT have arisen.[14-20]

Pfannenberg and colleagues[15] compared the low-dose nonenhanced CT and standard dose CECT in combined PET/CT protocols for staging and therapy planning in patients of non-small cell lung cancer (NSCLC). They concluded that in patients with advanced NSCLC, CECT as part of the PET/CT protocol was more accurate in assessing the TNM stage in around 8% of the patients as compared with noncontrast PET/CT. Most importantly for the radiotherapy and surgery planning, contrast-enhanced PET/CT proved to be indispensable owing to their precision in delineating the tumor. Similarly, contrast-enhanced PET/CT has been shown to be superior to nonenhanced PET/CT for preoperative nodal staging in rectal cancer,[16] for assessing the recurrence of ovarian cancer,[17] colorectal cancer,[18] and uterine cancer.[14]

A similar report of the superiority of contrast-enhanced PET/CT over noncontrast PET/CT was reported for assessing the resectability of pancreatic cancer.[19] Morimoto and colleagues[20] in their

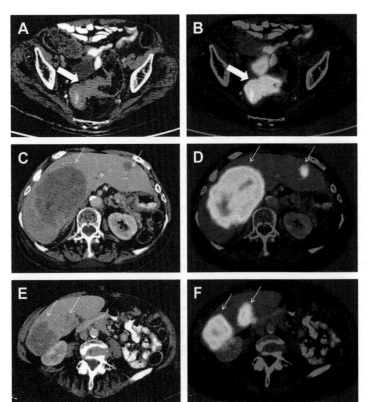

Fig. 1. An 80-year-old woman with carcinoma of the rectosigmoid junction underwent FDG PET/CT for staging. Axial CECT (*A, C, E*) and FDG PET/CT images (*B, D, F*) using intravenous and oral contrast completely delineate the primary as FDG avid (SUVmax, 13.04) circumferential wall thickening in the rectosigmoid junction (length 6.12 cm), with maximum wall thickness of 1.6 cm, causing significant luminal compromise (*A, B; bold white arrows*). Multiple FDG avid (SUVmax, 8.54), heterogeneously enhancing lesions with areas of central necrosis noted in both lobes of the liver (3 in right lobe, 1 in left lobe), largest in right lobe measuring 9.61 × 6.45 cm (*C–F; thin white arrows*). Note the well-distended bowel loops and well-delineated areas of necrosis in hepatic lesions as a result of the oral and intravenous contrast administration, respectively.

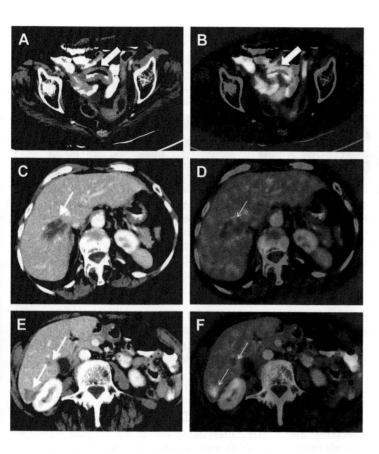

Fig. 2. Follow-up axial CECT (*A*, *C*, *E*) and FDG PET/CT images (*B*, *D*, *F*) of the patient in **Fig. 1** after undergoing palliative chemotherapy. It shows significant reduction in size and FDG avidity of the primary rectosigmoid mass (length 3.5 cm, SUVmax, 4.8) (*A*, *B*; *bold white arrows*) as well as the liver lesions (SUVmax, 2.6) (*C–F*; *thin white arrows*), which are well delineated by the use of oral and intravenous contrast administration, respectively, suggestive of significant response to treatment.

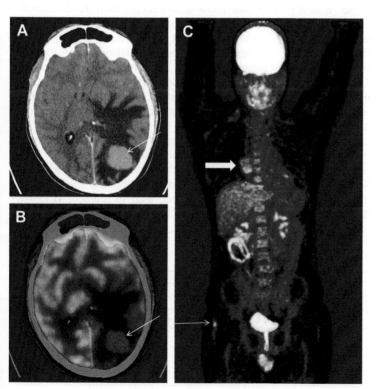

Fig. 3. A 36-year-old man with a space-occupying lesion (SOL) in the right parietal region was sent for FDG PET/CT for a whole-body workup. Axial CECT (*A*) and FDG PET/CT images (*B*) using intravenous contrast reveal a well-defined enhancing intra-axial SOL (2.2 × 2.5 cm) in left parietal lobe with minimal FDG avidity (SUVmax, 3.1). There is significant perilesional edema and mild midline shift toward the right (*A*, *B*; *thin white arrows*). Maximum intensity projection (MIP) PET image shows areas of increased radiotracer uptake in right hemithorax (paracardiac region) (*C*; *bold white arrow*) and right gluteal region (*C*; *thin white arrow*).

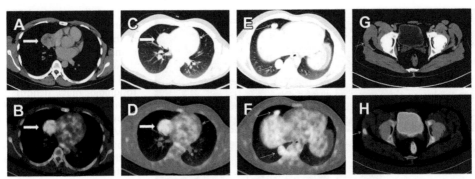

Fig. 4. Axial CT (*A, C, E, G*) and FDG PET/CT images (*B, D, F, H*) of the patient in **Fig. 3** reveals FDG avid (SUVmax, 7.39) soft tissue density mass (4.1 × 3.3 × 4.8 cm) in the right infrahilar region showing heterogeneous enhancement with areas of necrosis, which are better delineated using intravenous contrast (*A–D; bold white arrow*), likely indicative of primary pathologic abnormality with bilateral multiple pulmonary micronodular and macronodular lesions (*C–F; thin white arrows*). Also noted is focal FDG uptake in the right gluteus medius muscle (*G, H; thin white arrow*).

study of 66 patients with malignant lymphoma concluded that the contrast-enhanced PET/CT improves the diagnostic accuracy in evaluating nodal status (pelvic and retroperitoneal) in such patients.

The overestimation of PET attenuation factors as observed with the positive oral contrast agents is not a cause of concern with the use of intravenous contrast media in PET/CT because the contrast-related artifacts can be accurately attributed to the underlying vessels.[21] Mawlawi and colleagues[22] conducted a study to quantify the effect of intravenous contrast media in PET/CT and to assess its impact on patients with intrathoracic malignancies. They found that when CECT is used for attenuation correction, there is a corresponding increase in SUV in regions of high-contrast concentration, but the increase is clinically insignificant. Hence, they concluded that contrast-enhanced PET/CT can be used for the evaluation of patients with cancer.

Most of the intravenous contrast agents are usually based on iodine. These intravenous contrast agents are further classified into ionic (nonorganic) and nonionic (organic). Ionic agents were developed first, have higher osmolality, and have more side effects. Nonionic or organic agents, which covalently bind to iodine, are water soluble but do not dissociate, and hence, have lower osmolality and fewer side effects. **Tables 1** and **2** summarize the various ionic and nonionic contrast agents.[21,23]

Oral Contrast Agents

The 2 main categories of oral contrast agents are positive and negative agents. Positive contrast agents have a high atomic number and thus appear more radio-opaque than the surrounding tissue, for example, iodine and barium sulfate. Negative contrast agents have a lower atomic number and appear radiolucent, for example, gases (air, oxygen, carbon dioxide) and fluids (water, mannitol, sorbitol). Positive contrast materials increase the CT attenuation values of the bowel lumen, leading to its opacification and thus proper delineation from the adjacent structures (see **Figs. 1** and **2; Fig. 5**). Negative contrast agents ease image interpretation by causing bowel distension rather than opacification[21] (**Fig. 6**).

It has been recognized that the use of positive contrast agents can lead to artifacts in PET/CT arising from the CT-based attenuation correction of the PET images. Therefore, some centers avoid

Table 1
Commonly used iodinated (ionic) contrast agents

Compound Name	Type	Iodine Content (mg/mL)	Osmolality
Diatrizoate (Hypaque 50)	Monomer	300	1550 (High)
Metrizoate (Isopaque 370)	Monomer	370	2100 (High)
Ioxaglate (Hexabrix)	Dimer	320	580 (Low)

Table 2
Commonly used iodinated (nonionic) contrast agents

Compound Name	Type	Iodine Content (mg/mL)	Osmolality
Iopamidol (Isovue 370)	Monomer	370	796 (Low)
Iohexol (Omnipaque 350)	Monomer	350	884 (Low)
Ioxilan (Oxilan 350)	Monomer	350	695 (Low)
Iopromide (Ultravist 370)	Monomer	370	774 (Low)
Iodixanol (Visipaque 320)	Dimer	320	290 (Iso-osmolar)

the routine use of positive contrast agents, whereas others prefer using negative contrast agents.[24,25] A large prospective study was conducted by Groves and colleagues[26] on 200 patients to assess whether using positive oral contrast medium induces any artifacts of clinical relevance and whether these agents aid in diagnosis. Patients were administered 8 mL of gastrografin (sodium amidotrizoate 100 mg/mL, meglumine amidotrizoate 660 mg/mL, 370 mg I/mL, Schering Health Care, UK) in 500 mL of water (positive contrast) before PET/CT examination. They did not notice any positive oral contrast-induced artifacts of clinical significance. In addition to this, oral contrast agents aid in image interpretation by helping in differentiating a mass/node from bowel or intestinal wall from lumen. It is especially helpful in the region of the pancreatic bed, which is in close relationship with the duodenum and adjacent small bowel loops. However, whenever in doubt, nonattenuation corrected images should also be reviewed, because such PET images are free of contrast-related artifacts.[21]

Hence, the use of oral contrast medium in PET/CT is encouraged because it helps in proper delineation of the bowel loops without producing clinically significant artifacts and therefore improving image interpretation. Intestinal distension by the oral contrast agents helps in accurate assessment and extent of primary intestinal tumors and also of gut infiltration by the extraintestinal tumors. However, the use of oral contrast agents should be limited to patients in whom the site of suspected disease is in the gastrointestinal tract or abdomen. In other patients, for instance, head and neck malignancy, where abdominal disease is unlikely, the use of oral contrast agents is not justified. Moreover, it can lead to increased cervical muscle

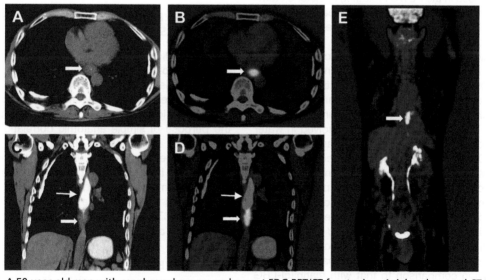

Fig. 5. A 50-year-old man with esophageal cancer underwent FDG PET/CT for staging. Axial and coronal CT (*A, C*) and FDG PET/CT images (*B, D*) reveal circumferential wall thickening extending for a length of 3.6 cm at the level of D9-10 vertebrae extending distally to just above the gastroesophageal junction, causing significant luminal compromise and showing increased FDG avidity (SUVmax, 7.56) (*A–E; bold white arrows*). Note the proximal esophageal dilatation and significant hold up of oral contrast (*C, D; thin white arrows*). MIP PET image (*E*) shows no evidence of distant disease.

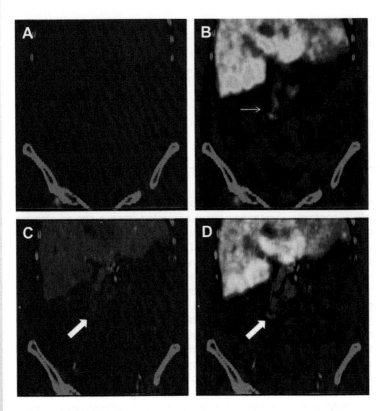

Fig. 6. Coronal CT (*A, C*) and ^{68}Ga-labeled [1,4,7,10-tetraaza-cyclododecane-1,4,7,10-tetraacetic acid]-1-NaI3-octreotide (DOTANOC) PET/CT images (*B, D*) in a patient with suspected neuroendocrine tumor. The upper row conventional CT (*A*) and PET/CT images (*B*) show mild and diffuse uptake of radiotracer in the duodenal area (*B; thin white arrow*). Lower row images (*C, D*) after giving intravenous and negative oral contrast show well-visualized area of focally increased tracer uptake in the second/third part of the duodenum corresponding to the focal nodular wall thickening on CT; likely indicative of primary pathologic abnormality (*C, D; bold white arrow*).

uptake in such patients, which can hamper image interpretation.[24]

Plain water is the simplest negative oral contrast agent used in the PET/CT imaging to distend stomach and bowel loops. However, it is easily absorbed in the bowel and can lead to variable and inconsistent bowel distension.[27] Another disadvantage with water is that it can induce a micturition urge if used in larger volumes, which can cause delay and interruption of PET/CT examination.[25]

Antoch and colleagues[25] compared a solution containing 0.2% locust bean gum (LBG) and 2.5% mannitol (mannitol-LBG) dissolved in water to provide a negative oral contrast material in PET/CT with oral barium (positive contrast agent) and water (negative contrast agent). Qualitative and quantitative analyses were performed for determining the effects of these contrast agents on bowel distention and influence on the PET data, if any. Mannitol-LBG provided the maximum bowel distention out of the 3 solutions. Increased FDG uptake was noted in the small bowel with barium in comparison to that with mannitol-LBG or water. They concluded that mannitol-LBG may be used as a negative oral contrast agent in PET/CT because it provides excellent bowel distention. Moreover, it also avoids the positive contrast material–induced PET artifacts (overestimation of

SUV). Other oral contrast agents that have been tried in the past include whole (4%) milk, 2% milk,[28] and polyethylene glycol.[29]

CONTRAST PET/COMPUTED TOMOGRAPHY PROTOCOLS

As the application of CECT in PET/CT started growing, efforts were made to optimize the imaging protocols. In general, 2 main protocols are being followed all over the world. In one protocol, nondiagnostic low-dose CT is done, mainly for the purpose of simple anatomic correlation and attenuation correction of PET images. Oral contrast agents may be used depending on the clinical indication. In the second protocol, full-dose contrast-enhanced diagnostic CT is acquired, thus minimizing the need for additional diagnostic CTs.[21,30] Both the protocols are summarized in **Table 3**.

ADVERSE REACTIONS TO CONTRAST AGENTS

Detailed history of each patient should be taken to rule out any contraindication for the use of contrast media. Risk factors include a history of previous allergy-like reaction to the contrast media. Such patients have a 5-fold increased likelihood

Table 3
Imaging protocols in PET/computed tomography

Protocol	CT	Purpose of CT	Contrast Agents	Radiation Dose	Need for Additional Diagnostic CTs
1.	Nondiagnostic	• Attenuation correction of PET images • Simple anatomic correlation with PET	Usually oral for bowel delineation	Low	Yes
2.	State-of-the-art diagnostic CT	• Excellent information on anatomy and tumor vascularization • Attenuation correction of PET images	Usually both oral and intravenous	High	No

of experiencing a subsequent reaction.[31] Also, patients with significant allergies, like a major anaphylactic response to any allergen in the past, need special attention. Atopic patients with a history of allergy to food products (eg, dairy products) are also at a 2 to 3 times increased risk for a contrast reaction.[32] Patients with asthma or multiple myeloma and those with renal insufficiency are also at increased risk of contrast reaction.[23,33]

Severity of Reaction

From a clinical point of view, contrast reactions may be divided into mild, moderate, and severe. Mild reactions are the most common and include itching, flushing, pallor, rashes, and so on and usually require observation and reassurance. Moderate reactions like tachycardia, hypotension,

bronchospasm, laryngeal edema, and others require prompt treatment and close observation. Rarely, severe, life-threatening reactions may occur like progressive laryngeal edema, profound hypotension, cardiopulmonary arrest, convulsions, and so on that require hospitalization and prompt intervention.[1,21]

CONTRAST-BASED SPECIAL TECHNIQUES IN PET/COMPUTED TOMOGRAPHY
PET/Computed Tomography Enteroclysis

CT enteroclysis is a specialized technique that involves an abdominal CT after fluoroscopic intubation infusion of small bowel with a contrast agent. It provides excellent anatomic information regarding mucosal abnormalities, bowel thickening, fistulae, lower grades of bowel obstruction,

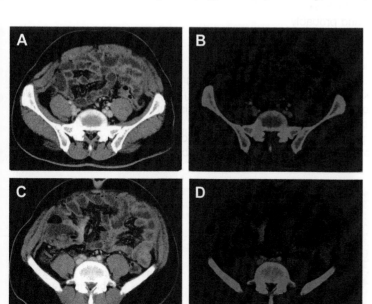

Fig. 7. Normal FDG PET/CT enteroclysis study. Axial CT (*A, C*) and FDG PET/CT images (*B, D*) after luminal distension demonstrate prominent and better delineated small-bowel loops with no abnormal area of radiotracer uptake.

adhesions, and so on.[34] However, it fails to show the metabolic activity of the disease.

Das and colleagues[35] conceptualized a novel method of fusing metabolic imaging technique (PET) with an anatomic imaging modality (CT enteroclysis). In their prospective study on 17 patients with newly diagnosed inflammatory diseases of the intestine, PET/CT enteroclysis of the abdomen was performed after infusion of 2 L of 0.5% methylcellulose through a nasojejunal catheter. The motive was to derive information on morphology and functional activity of lesions at the same time. They found that PET/CT enteroclysis detects a significantly higher number of lesions in the bowel (small and large intestine) as compared with conventional barium and colonoscopy studies combined. Hence, they concluded that PET/CT enteroclysis is a noninvasive, feasible, and very promising tool for the evaluation of inflammatory diseases of the intestine. Detailed techniques have been described by Das and colleagues[36] (Fig. 7).

Diuretic Fluorodeoxyglucose PET/Computed Tomography Scan

Diuretic FDG PET/CT works on the principle of replacing radioactive urine in the bladder with non-radioactive urine (a negative contrast agent) within a permissible timespan (before significant biological decay of ^{18}F-FDG) by using the special technique of forced diuresis (Fig. 8). FDG PET/CT has been used earlier for staging of patients with carcinoma bladder, but the results were not promising[37–39] due to the fact that ^{18}F-FDG is excreted through the urinary tract, which leads to masking of the primary lesion in the bladder and probably perivesical lymph nodes as well.[39] The role of FDG PET/CT in such patients was limited to the detection of regional lymph nodes and distant metastases.[37]

Therefore, an intervention to reduce the ^{18}F-FDG activity in the urine was required without altering the ^{18}F-FDG uptake in the primary tumor. Nayak and colleagues[40] developed a novel method to overcome this limitation. They used furosemide, a loop diuretic, to enhance the renal elimination of the excreted ^{18}F-FDG without altering its uptake in the primary vesical tumor. Furosemide allowed a sufficient time window for the reduction of ^{18}F-FDG activity in the bladder, before any significant biologic decay of ^{18}F-FDG has occurred.

Nayak and colleagues[40] prospectively evaluated 25 patients with suspected primary carcinoma of the urinary bladder who underwent conventional CECT of the abdomen/pelvis and whole-body diuretic FDG PET/CT for the purpose of diagnosis and staging. Apart from the whole-body PET/CT images (skull base to mid thigh), pelvic PET/CT images were acquired after forced diuresis with intravenous furosemide (20–40 mg). Subsequently, 10 patients underwent radical cystectomy and 15 underwent transurethral resection of the bladder tumor.

Thereafter, the results of CECT and diuretic FDG PET/CT were compared with histopathology as a reference standard. FDG PET/CT was found to be superior to CECT in the detection of the primary tumor as well as for the locoregional staging ($P<.05$). Similar promising results were shown by Anjos and colleagues,[41] who in their study on 17 patients with bladder cancer found that the detection of locally recurrent or residual bladder tumors can be dramatically improved using FDG PET/CT with delayed images after diuretic and oral hydration. Not only bladder carcinoma but also diuretic FDG PET/CT has been shown to improve evaluation of FDG activity and extent of tumor in other pelvic malignancies like carcinoma cervix.[42]

SUMMARY

To conclude, the state-of-the-art contrast-enhanced diagnostic PET/CT is here to stay, looks promising, and not only provides excellent anatomic details but also information on tumor vascularization as well. Moreover, the need for additional diagnostic imaging modalities is reduced, thereby saving time, which may have

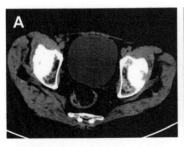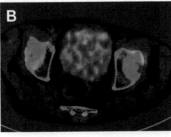

Fig. 8. After diuretic axial CT (A) and FDG PET/CT images (B) in a follow-up case of carcinoma bladder who underwent transurethral resection of the bladder tumor show a well-distended bladder with minimal FDG activity and no significant area of abnormal radiotracer uptake.

an important bearing on the patient management and clinical outcome.

REFERENCES

1. American College of Radiology Committee on Drugs and Contrast Media. ACR manual on contrast media. 9th edition. Reston (VA): American College of Radiology; 2013. p. 4–11.
2. Kapoor V, McCook BM, Torok FS. An introduction to PET-CT imaging. RadioGraphics 2004;24:523–43.
3. Phelps ME. PET: the merging of biology and imaging into molecular imaging. J Nucl Med 2000;41:661–81.
4. Goerres GW, Stupp R, Barghouth G, et al. The value of PET, CT and in-line PET-CT in patients with gastrointestinal stromal tumors: long-term outcome of treatment with imatinib mesylate. Eur J Nucl Med Mol Imaging 2005;32:153–62.
5. Dhull VS, Sharma P, Sharma DN, et al. Prospective evaluation of 18F fluorodeoxyglucose positron emission tomography-computed tomography for response evaluation in recurrent carcinoma cervix: does metabolic response predicts survival? Int J Gynecol Cancer 2014;24:312–20.
6. Antoch G, Saoudi N, Kuehl H, et al. Accuracy of whole-body dual-modality FDG-PET/CT for tumor staging in oncology: comparison with CT and PET. J Clin Oncol 2004;22:4357–68.
7. Yoshida K, Suzuki A, Nagashima T, et al. Staging primary head and neck cancers with (18)F-FDG PET/CT: is intravenous contrast administration really necessary? Eur J Nucl Med Mol Imaging 2009;36:1417–24.
8. Kuehl H, Antoch G. How much CT do we need for PET/CT? A radiologist's perspective. Nuklearmedizin 2005;44:S24–31.
9. Strobel K, Thuerl CM, Hany TF. How much intravenous contrast is needed in FDG-PET/CT? Nuklearmedizin 2005;44:S32–7.
10. Schaefer NG, Hany TF, Taverna C, et al. Non-Hodgkin lymphoma and Hodgkin disease: coregistered FDG-PET and CT at staging and restaging – do we need contrast-enhanced CT? Radiology 2004;232:823–9.
11. Coleman RE, Delbeke D, Guiberteau MJ, et al. Concurrent PET/CT with an integrated imaging system: intersociety dialogue from the joint working group of the American College of Radiology, the Society of Nuclear Medicine, and the Society of Computed Body Tomography and Magnetic Resonance. J Nucl Med 2005;46:1225–39.
12. Pfannenberg AC, Aschoff P, Brechtel K, et al. Value of contrast-enhanced multiphase CT in combined PET/CT protocols for oncological imaging. Br J Radiol 2007;80:437–45.
13. Antoch G, Freudenberg LS, Beyer T, et al. To enhance or not to enhance? 18F-FDG and CT contrast agents in dual-modality 18F-FDG PET/CT. J Nucl Med 2004;45:56S–65S.
14. Kitajima K, Suzuki K, Nakamoto Y, et al. Low-dose non-enhanced CT versus full-dose contrast-enhanced CT in integrated PET/CT studies for the diagnosis of uterine cancer recurrence. Eur J Nucl Med Mol Imaging 2010;37:1490–8.
15. Pfannenberg AC, Aschoff P, Brechtel K, et al. Low dose non-enhanced CT versus standard dose contrast-enhanced CT in combined PET/CT protocols for staging and therapy planning in non-small cell lung cancer. Eur J Nucl Med Mol Imaging 2007;34:36–44.
16. Tateishi U, Maeda T, Morimoto T, et al. Non-enhanced CT versus contrast-enhanced CT in integrated PET/CT studies for nodal staging of rectal cancer. Eur J Nucl Med Mol Imaging 2007;34:1627–34.
17. Kitajima K, Murakami K, Yamasaki E, et al. Performance of integrated FDG-PET/contrast-enhanced CT in the diagnosis of recurrent ovarian cancer: comparison with integrated FDG-PET/non-contrast-enhanced CT and enhanced CT. Eur J Nucl Med Mol Imaging 2008;35:1439–48.
18. Kitajima K, Murakami K, Yamasaki E, et al. Performance of integrated FDG-PET/contrast-enhanced CT in the diagnosis of recurrent colorectal cancer: comparison with integrated FDG-PET/non-contrast-enhanced CT and enhanced CT. Eur J Nucl Med Mol Imaging 2009;36:1388–96.
19. Strobel K, Heinrich S, Bhure U, et al. Contrast-enhanced 18F-FDG PET/CT: 1-stop-shop imaging for assessing the respectability of pancreatic cancer. J Nucl Med 2008;49:1408–13.
20. Morimoto T, Tateishi U, Maeda T, et al. Nodal status of malignant lymphoma in pelvic and retroperitoneal lymphatic pathways: comparison of integrated PET/CT with or without contrast enhancement. Eur J Radiol 2008;67:508–13.
21. Antoch G, Veit P, Bockisch A, et al. Application of CT Contrast Agents in PET-CT Imaging. In: Shreve P, Townsend DW, editors. Clinical PET-CT in radiology: integrated imaging in oncology. New York: Springer; 2010. p. 91–101.
22. Mawlawi O, Erasmus JJ, Munden RF, et al. Quantifying the effect of IV contrast media on integrated PET/CT: clinical evaluation. AJR Am J Roentgenol 2006;186:308–19.
23. Singh J, Daftary A. Iodinated contrast media and their adverse reactions. J Nucl Med Technol 2008;36:69–74.
24. Cohade C, Osman M, Nakamoto Y, et al. Initial experience with oral contrast in PET/CT: phantom and clinical studies. J Nucl Med 2003;44:412–6.
25. Antoch G, Kuehl H, Kanja J, et al. Dual-modality PET/CT scanning with negative oral contrast agent to avoid artifacts: introduction and evaluation. Radiology 2004;230:879–85.

26. Groves AM, Kayani I, Dickson JC, et al. Oral contrast medium in PET/CT: should you or shouldn't you? Eur J Nucl Med Mol Imaging 2005;32:1160–6.

27. Winter TC, Ager JD, Nghiem HV, et al. Upper gastro-intestinal tract and abdomen: water as an orally administered contrast agent for helical CT. Radiology 1996;201:365–70.

28. Thompson SE, Raptopoulos V, Sheiman RL, et al. Abdominal helical CT: milk as a low-attenuation oral contrast agent. Radiology 1999;211:870–5.

29. Hebert JJ, Taylor AJ, Winter TC, et al. Low-attenuation oral GI contrast agents in abdominal-pelvic computed tomography. Abdom Imaging 2006;31:48–53.

30. Beyer T, Antoch G, Müller S, et al. Acquisition protocol considerations for combined PET/CT imaging. J Nucl Med 2004;45:25S–35S.

31. Katayama H, Yamaguchi K, Kozuka T, et al. Adverse reactions to ionic and nonionic contrast media. A report from the Japanese Committee on the Safety of Contrast Media. Radiology 1990;175:621–8.

32. Coakley FV, Panicek DM. Iodine allergy: an oyster without a pearl? AJR Am J Roentgenol 1997;169:951–2.

33. Katzberg RW. Urography into the 21st century: new contrast media, renal handling, imaging characteristics, and nephrotoxicity. Radiology 1997;204:297–312.

34. Maglinte DD, Sandrasegaran K, Lappas JC, et al. CT enteroclysis. Radiology 2007;245:661–71.

35. Das CJ, Makharia G, Kumar R, et al. PET-CT enteroclysis: a new technique for evaluation of inflammatory diseases of the intestine. Eur J Nucl Med Mol Imaging 2007;34:2106–14.

36. Das CJ. PET/CT enteroclysis. PET Clin 2016, in press.

37. Kibel AS, Dehdashti F, Katz MD, et al. Prospective study of [18F]fluorodeoxyglucose positron emission tomography/computed tomography for staging of muscle-invasive bladder carcinoma. J Clin Oncol 2009;27:4314–20.

38. Apolo AB, Riches J, Schöder H, et al. Clinical value of fluorine-18 2-fluoro-2-deoxy-D-glucose positron emission tomography/computed tomography in bladder cancer. J Clin Oncol 2010;28:3973–8.

39. Drieskens O, Oyen R, Van Poppel H, et al. FDG-PET for preoperative staging of bladder cancer. Eur J Nucl Med Mol Imaging 2005;32:1412–7.

40. Nayak B, Dogra PN, Naswa N, et al. Diuretic 18F-FDG PET/CT imaging for detection and locoregional staging of urinary bladder cancer: prospective evaluation of a novel technique. Eur J Nucl Med Mol Imaging 2013;40:386–93.

41. Anjos DA, Etchebehere ECSC, Ramos CD, et al. 18F-FDG PET/CT delayed images after diuretic for restaging invasive bladder cancer. J Nucl Med 2007;48:764–70.

42. d'Amico A, Gorczewska I, Gorczewski K, et al. Effect of furosemide administration before F-18 fluorodeoxyglucose positron emission tomography/computed tomography on urine radioactivity and detection of uterine cervical cancer. Nucl Med Rev Cent East Eur 2014;17:83–6.

Moving?

Make sure your subscription moves with you!

To notify us of your new address, find your **Clinics Account Number** (located on your mailing label above your name), and contact customer service at:

Email: journalscustomerservice-usa@elsevier.com

800-654-2452 (subscribers in the U.S. & Canada)
314-447-8871 (subscribers outside of the U.S. & Canada)

Fax number: 314-447-8029

Elsevier Health Sciences Division
Subscription Customer Service
3251 Riverport Lane
Maryland Heights, MO 63043

ELSEVIER

Printed and bound by CPI Group (UK) Ltd, Croydon, CR0 4YY

03/10/2024

01040377-0004